CO ARSENIC
IN THE
Dumplings

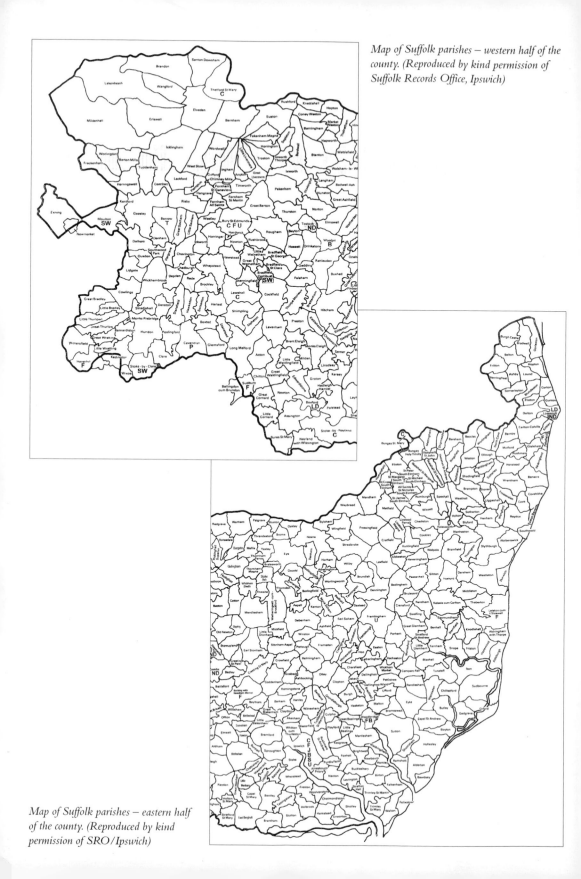

Map of Suffolk parishes – western half of the county. (Reproduced by kind permission of Suffolk Records Office, Ipswich)

Map of Suffolk parishes – eastern half of the county. (Reproduced by kind permission of SRO / Ipswich)

ARSENIC

IN THE

Dumplings

A Casebook of Historic Poisonings in Suffolk

SHEILA HARDY

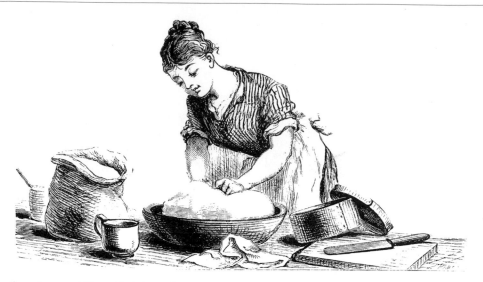

Arsenic: n.   (Chem.) brittle steel-grey semi-metallic substance, crystallizing in rhombohedrons, & volatising without fusion with odour of garlic; (pop.) tri-oxide of ~, white mineral substance, a violent poison. (*Concise Oxford Dictionary*)

Traditional Recipe for Suffolk Dumplings
½ lb Flour
tsp Salt
Water to mix

Mix water into flour and salt to form a dough. Divide into small balls. Place into boiling water in the copper or a pan over the fire for twenty minutes or so.
May be added to stew of boiled mutton or to a broth.
Larger dumplings may be steamed in a cloth.

First published 2010

The History Press
The Mill, Brimscombe Port
Stroud, Gloucestershire, GL5 2QG
www.thehistorypress.co.uk

ISBN 978 0 7524 5132 9

Typesetting and origination by The History Press
Printed in India, Aegean Offset
Manufacturing managed by Jellyfish Print Solutions Ltd

CONTENTS

Acknowledgements   6

Introduction   7

one   Elizabeth Wooltorton, North Cove, 1815   13

two   Elizabeth Gooch, Bruisyard, 1835   19

three   John Bartram, Gislingham, 1835   26

four   Mary Sheming, Martlesham, 1845   32

five   Catharine Foster, Acton, 1847   41

six   Mary Cage, Stonham Aspal, 1851   54

seven   William Rowlinson, Great Thurlow, 1851   66

eight   William Baldry, Preston, 1851   73

nine   Letitia Newman, Laxfield, 1863   80

ten   The Silver Family, Rickinghall, 1865   86

Appendix: Mr Clubbe's Accounts   92

Sources   95

ACKNOWLEDGEMENTS

I wish to offer my most sincere thanks to the following for their help with my research: Mr and Mrs Peter Atkins; Mary Bray; Sharon Miller, Waldringfield Baptist Church; The White Horse Inn, Badingham; Ray Wright.

As on previous occasions Patricia Burnham generously shared her great genealogical knowledge; Dr E. Cockayne readily answered my often peculiar queries on medical matters, and Sue Kerswell proofread the manuscript. Roger Lane of Acton showed great kindness in allowing me the use of photographs from his archive. The enthusiastic staff at the Register Offices in Ipswich and Sudbury were most helpful and encouraging, as were the staff at all three Suffolk Records Offices. A special thank you to Sarah Steggles and Katie Vaughan of the Bury Record Office for their exceptional kindness.

And finally to Michael, who not only willingly ferried me around Suffolk to find the location of these cases and took all the photographs but also continued to eat my cooking – even stew with dumplings!

INTRODUCTION

Even today, at the beginning of the twenty-first century, it is possible to recapture a sense of what Suffolk must have been like 200 years ago. Take a turning off one of the three main roads that radiate from Ipswich, already established as an important trading centre long before medieval times, and you will find yourself driving through narrow roads that follow the line of field patterns laid down centuries ago. Long before the huge prairie-type fields that make East Anglia the bread-basket of the United Kingdom were created, small fields surrounded the villages, many of them monastic holdings where the labourers practised the three-field method of farming that supported the local population. Suffolk's main product then was not its golden wheat but its golden fleece. The conditions which provided lush pasture, quickly made the county the centre of the wool-producing business, which expanded and grew into a major industry throughout the Middle Ages and right up to the early eighteenth century.

The wealth that flowed from wool manufacture is still visible today in some of the tiniest villages, where a magnificent flint church, seemingly far too big for a rural area, is the legacy of the local merchants who once owned the land and gave the money to build these fine old buildings. Often too, we can find other traces of their largesse in the quaint old almshouses, but a lasting testimony to the importance of the wool trade remains in the number of substantially built, thatched, timber-framed houses in the many small market towns that grew up throughout the county, some of which still retain their old Guildhalls. Lavenham is perhaps the best-known example, but there are countless gems to be found in the most unexpected places.

There are many reasons for the decline of the trade in Suffolk, the most obvious being the development of machinery to do the work of spinning and weaving and related trades such as fulling and dyeing. This had a disastrous impact on the livelihood of agricultural labourers who, by cottage industry, supplemented their incomes, particularly in winter. A spinning wheel was often the most important item in the house: both the raw material and the finished product were delivered and collected by the wool merchant's itinerant travellers. Whole families were involved in the work, including the children, who knitted stockings. Much of this came to an end when factories were able to turn out products at a

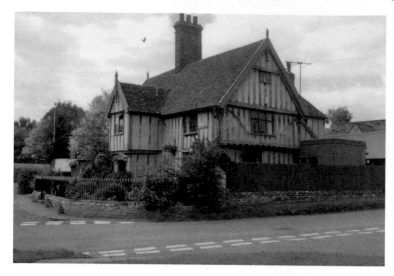

A Suffolk timber-framed house. (Author's collection)

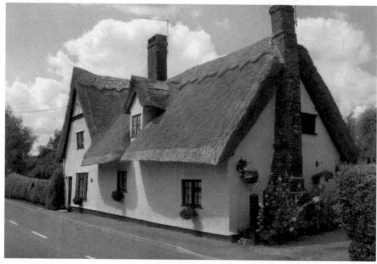

A Suffolk thatched cottage. (Author's collection)

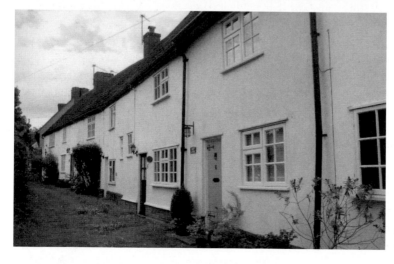

Terrace of eighteenth-century cottages. (Author's collection)

quicker and more economical rate. Landowners found they could make bigger profits with large flocks of sheep to supply the factories. So they enclosed their land, thus changing the pattern of farming – as the nursery rhyme tells us, 'the cows in the meadow, the sheep in the corn' – and taking in too the common land that for centuries had given the labourer the right to gather firewood, graze his animals and let his pigs forage in the woodlands. Instead he was limited to the small piece of ground around the homestead in which he lived, courtesy of his employer. However, if that employer, often an absentee, was now using his land solely for sheep, then the numbers of men he employed were seriously depleted and the labourer could find himself not only jobless, but homeless too.

The effect of this was twofold, the young and those who could, left the countryside and migrated to the towns to find work, many making the journey north to the factories. But for those who remained, their standard of living was reduced greatly, and they were often faced with such poverty that they were forced to seek the assistance of Parish Relief. The system introduced in Elizabethan times where each English parish undertook to look after those in need within its boundaries had worked well. Everyone within the parish who owned property over a certain value was charged an annual percentage of that value to fund the income necessary to provide for its poor and needy residents. Known as the Poor Rate, it was administered by the Overseers of the Poor, who were elected each year at the annual Parish Meeting, at which the year's rate was set and decisions made as to how much should be paid out for different circumstances.

While the economy of the country as a whole was flourishing, the system worked well, business people and those with private incomes could well afford their contributions but as entries in the old Suffolk Rate Books show, by the mid-1700s many of these had fallen on hard times themselves and were unable to meet their commitments. Previously, every parish had had a house set aside to provide temporary shelter for the homeless or those too old to work, but with rising unemployment new ways had to be devised to deal with the growing poverty. A new Poor Law was introduced and with it came the building of huge workhouses designed to provide both accommodation and work for the unemployed.

Towns probably fared better than villages, where there were fewer affluent householders and businesses to make contributions, yet it was here that the need was greatest. Absentee landlords often failed to repair their property, or in an attempt to make more profit gave orders that existing double tenements be subdivided to form three or four homes. Today, when we look at the carefully restored, picturesque sixteenth-century cottages that abound throughout the county, it is difficult to imagine what the home of the average labourer was like. Thatched, yes, but very roughly so in comparison with today's manicured roof. Most likely it was a single-storey dwelling with a ladder up to the roof, turning the space into a makeshift bedroom. In double, triple or even quadruple blocks, the lofts were intercommunicating, which at times may have put an interesting slant on having a close relationship with ones neighbours!

The actual construction of the building was of lath interspersed with material which might be animal dung, horsehair or whatever else happened to be at hand, overlaid with plaster that was then lime-washed both inside and out. The interior was painted white while Suffolk developed its own distinctive look for the exterior. Proudly boasting that every part of the pig had its use, its blood was mixed to the wash to achieve 'Suffolk pink', in fact a much darker shade than its name suggests. The floor might be flagged but more likely it was simply trodden solid with usage and possibly covered with straw or reeds. Although these might be changed regularly, they were an ideal breeding ground for insects and vermin and could also encourage dampness. Furniture was minimal, a table or a board placed upon a simple trestle, a few stools and roughly-made wooden chests to house flour and other dry stores. Extra clothes could also be stored in chests, which doubled as additional seating. If the room had a wide hearth then it was possible that part of the area at the side of it was raised up to form the basis of a bed. Parents and younger children usually occupied this; the older ones occupying the loft space, sleeping on mattresses made from straw-filled ticking. Refinements such as sheets and coverlets depended very much on the financial position of the family. Every bride hoped that she would have enough household items laid by ready for her marriage, but in an age when items were hand-made and expensive it was not uncommon for families to pass on their household goods and indeed their clothes. Shakespeare was not insulting his wife when he willed her his second-best bed; the best one automatically went with his house to his heir. Two hundred years later, anyone with sufficient property to leave made sure that 'my household furniture, linen, plate, goods chattels and effects ...' was duly given to someone who would make use of it or might have need of it.

Family historians often wonder how all the children of their eighteenth and nineteenth-century ancestors managed to cram into such overcrowded surroundings. The answer is that they often did not. Working life started very young, so girls frequently became servants as early as eleven or twelve. And because it was common practice for maidservants to live-in with their employers, this relieved pressure on parents who no longer had to feed them, and also freed up space for younger members of the family. Boys too, often lived on the farms where they worked, or in the home of their master if they were apprenticed to a tradesman. If older working children were not offered living accommodation with their job, then it was likely they might be lodged with elderly relations. That had a twofold advantage; the overcrowding in their own home was relieved while the elderly received a boost to their income.

As will become apparent in some of the cases that follow, domestic life was very basic. The main room of the house was both a living room and kitchen. Cooking was mainly over an open fire and thus limited to dishes that could be boiled. Lucky were those with bread ovens. Water for drinking and washing was supplied either from a communal well, often some distance from the house, or from a nearby pond or stream. Both sources were liable to fluctuation and contamination. Raw sewage and household rubbish were simply thrown on to a midden-heap away from the cottage, perhaps close to a hedge. Seepage from this, particularly after rain, would leak into the ditch that ran into the stream which provided the water supply. Under these conditions, it was no wonder that during the summer months in particular, there were serious outbreaks of 'the English Cholera' that would require medical attention.

During the eighteenth and early nineteenth centuries there was a strong division between the two main branches of the medical profession. Sons of gentlemen, landowners and the more wealthy clergy studied medicine at one of the great universities and, having gained the degree of MD, earned the right to call themselves 'doctor'. They then became known as physicians and were likely to practise in towns and cities with a wealthy patient list. A surgeon, on the other hand, learned his craft as an apprentice to an established surgeon. This branch of medicine had grown from the barber-surgeons and apothecaries who dispensed drugs. So the surgeon was not only a general practitioner, he could also perform operations and dispense medicine. The medical practitioners who were employed under the Poor Law were almost always surgeons and were always referred to as 'Mister', not doctor.

A labourer, unable to pay the surgeon himself, would have to first seek the necessary form from the local Relieving Officer. Armed with this he would then set out to walk, usually to

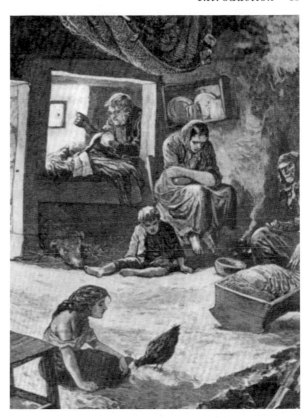

Cottage interior. (Reproduced from Looking Back, *by Philip Sauvain)*

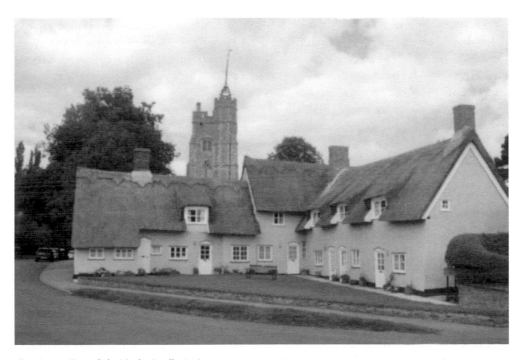

Cottages at Cavendish. (Author's collection)

the nearest town, to consult the surgeon and perhaps ask for a visit to the sick. Hours might pass before a patient was seen. Sometimes, having listened to the symptoms, rather than making a visit, the surgeon would send a basic medicine, usually an indigestion mixture or purgative. When the same symptoms presented at certain times of the year, it was not surprising that medical men might occasionally make the wrong diagnosis in a case. This was especially so where severe illness or even death was due to the ingestion of arsenic.

Arsenic in small doses was not lethal; the medical profession used it as a treatment for syphilis and gout, for example, while a restorative tonic containing arsenic was often prescribed for young ladies who were losing weight and lacking energy. Since arsenic is a natural substance it can be found all around us in the ground and in water supplies. But in its powdered form it was the recognised way to exterminate the rats and mice which regularly infested homes as well as barns and other outbuildings where food was stored. Small amounts could be readily bought in the local shop where the customers were known to the shopkeeper. It was also widely used in animal husbandry in preparations such as sheep dip to kill off insect infestations on a sheep's fleece. We also learn from some of the cases that follow that cereal farmers steeped their seed in a solution of arsenic to prevent insect attack during germination. That arsenic appears to be the poison favoured for premeditated murder in the eighteenth and nineteenth centuries was due solely to its general availability, especially in rural areas.

It is said that poison is a woman's weapon of choice, and indeed in the cases recorded here only three men were accused of using arsenic with intent to kill. This is obviously because poison can be placed in food and since it was usually women who prepared and cooked meals the opportunity was there. During the first half of the nineteenth century it was noted throughout the country that the number of women whose husbands had died in suspicious circumstances had risen rapidly. This may account for why women were treated far more severely when they came to trial and also why it was necessary for Parliament to introduce stringent regulations with regard to the sale of poisons.

The symptoms of arsenic poisoning included vomiting, diarrhoea, stomach cramps, excessive sweating, thirst and problems with swallowing. Since all these could also apply to the English Cholera, it became essential when death followed these symptoms to be able to discount the presence of arsenic in the body. So it was that we witness the development of what we now know as forensic science. Throughout these pages there will be many references to Mr Image, the doctor in Bury St Edmunds who made a name for himself as an expert witness in suspected murder cases. As the century progressed, so too did the experiments to ascertain the accuracy of the presence of arsenic. What is also fascinating is the graphic detail of post-mortem examinations and laboratory tests which were not only given in evidence but were also minutely reported in the local newspapers. We who avidly watch television dramas have become inured to seeing corpses dissected on mortuary slabs, their vital organs being placed by bloody hands in a scale pan. The Victorian journalist had to rely on words to create his impact. You must judge for yourself how successful he was.

Sheila Hardy, 2010

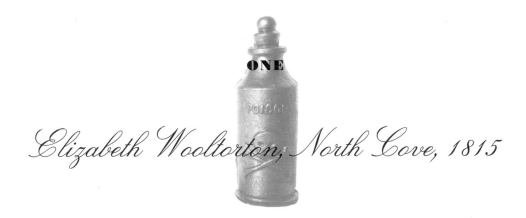

Elizabeth Wooltorton, North Cove, 1815

It might seem somewhat strange to start a history of Suffolk poisonings with an account of the events surrounding a woman whose address was actually in Norfolk. The excuse is that her home lay very close to the county boundary and that both her intended and actual victims were living in Suffolk. And, it has to be said that although the details are meagre, the case of Elizabeth Wooltorton makes a refreshing change from most of the other cases that follow in so far as Elizabeth came from yeoman rather than peasant stock.

At the time she came to public attention in July 1815, Elizabeth was a widow in her late forties. She and her late husband James had farmed in the village of Denton. They had had nine children, one of whom, a son probably born in 1805, had been given the name of the great naval hero, Nelson. The admiral had particular significance for them, for not only was he a Norfolk man, he also had connections with the village of Woolterton, from which the family had derived its surname. James, it would appear, was not a very astute businessman and some years before, when he was in the milling trade, he had gone bankrupt. It is possible that it was after this that they had borrowed £200 from James's wealthy uncle, Tifford Clarke, to enable them to rent the farm in Denton.

Neither the term of the loan nor the amount of interest Clarke expected is known, but whatever they were weighed heavily on Elizabeth's mind. Only one event could extricate her from both repayment of the principal and the overdue interest, and that was the death of Clarke, for he had promised to leave his nephew the Swan Inn and its surrounding land in Kirby Cane. The property currently brought Clarke a good rent from its tenant and as a legacy was reckoned to be worth in the region of £500. As Clarke was then in his eighties, there was a reasonable chance that Elizabeth and her family would not have to wait too long for their inheritance.

Tifford Clarke was a man of substance with sufficient wealth and status to be accorded the title of 'gentleman'. He owned considerable land let out as farms, as well as various properties that had outbuildings and land. The extent of his holdings was shown by the fact that he had made several successful petitions to Parliament to enclose land under the Act of Enclosure, land that straddled both sides of the county border – and he was still adding to his property portfolio.

Clarke, who had neither a wife nor any immediate family, did have a cousin, Mrs Mary Pleasants, who acted as his housekeeper. She obviously looked after him well, not only

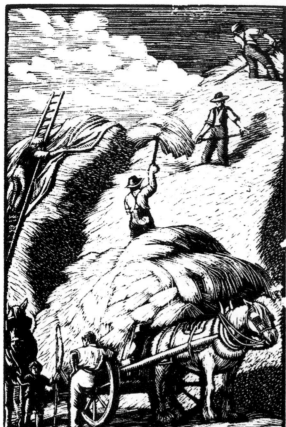

Haymaking. (Reproduced by kind permission of the Foxearth & District History Society)

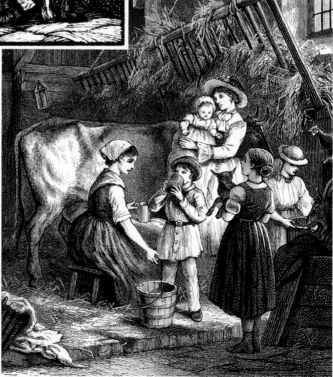

Milking. *Taken from* The Infant's Magazine *for 1887.* *(Author's collection)*

running the house smoothly and making sure that he had only the best quality food; she also shielded him from unwanted callers. Thanks to her care he was still very active in both body and mind. However, while others may have rejoiced at the gentleman's good health and longevity, Elizabeth, whose financial situation was worsening, decided that the time had come to lend nature a helping hand. So, on at least two occasions while baking, she made an extra cake, later alleged to contain the additional ingredient of arsenic, and sent them to Clarke. He, having suffered a slight stomach upset after eating a piece of the first cake, thanked Elizabeth politely for her kind thought, but, reminding her of the precarious state of her family's financial position, requested that she should refrain from sending him gifts.

Undeterred by this, Elizabeth bided her time before sending another present. On that occasion a pie and a piece of veal accompanied the cake. Doubt exists as to who did the actual baking. Elizabeth was to maintain that she asked her daughter, Amy, to make the cake and pie, while Amy insisted that her part was merely to follow her mother's instructions to pack the items in a basket and make sure that it was delivered to Tifford Clarke's house.

Young Nelson Wooltorton set out at six o'clock on the morning of Sunday 2 July to walk the six miles or so from Denton to Kirby Cane. When he arrived at about ten o'clock Mrs Pleasants received him in the kitchen, where she unpacked the basket. No doubt she offered the lad some refreshment before he started on his return journey, but he did not appear to have had any contact with Mr Clarke.

Presumably Mrs Pleasants had been made aware of Clarke's feelings about gifts from the Wooltortons, but rather than offend Elizabeth by refusing them, she felt justified in passing on at least one of the items. It was never revealed what happened to the joint of meat or the pie, but the cake she wrapped up and gave to her son-in-law, Benjamin Sparkes, when he called on her later that day. As a farm labourer, Benjamin was always glad of the little luxuries that his mother-in-law was able to give them so he carried the cake home to his village of North Cove knowing it would be most welcomed by his wife Sarah and their children. It was late when he got home and everyone was asleep, so he left the cake on the table before climbing into bed beside his wife. The next day, Monday, Benjamin left for work at six and after he had gone, Sarah prepared the usual breakfast of bread and butter for the children. Today, however, they were to have an additional treat – the cake grandmother had sent them. This was carefully cut into a dozen or more equal slices. Like her husband, Sarah was going to be working that day in the hayfields so she had arranged with her neighbour, Mrs Mills, to come in to supervise breakfast, make sure that the older children got off to school on time and remain with the younger ones until her return. Mrs Mills brought her young family with her. Before she left, Sarah showed Mrs Mills the cake and told her that she and her children were very welcome to share it.

After a couple of hours of gathering the hay into sheaves, Sarah returned to the cottage for her breakfast. She was totally unprepared for the scene that greeted her. Instead of an almost empty house she found that Mrs Mills and four of her children had all been violently sick, while her five-year-old son, Robert, was apparently having convulsions. She had barely got through the door when two more of her children started to vomit.

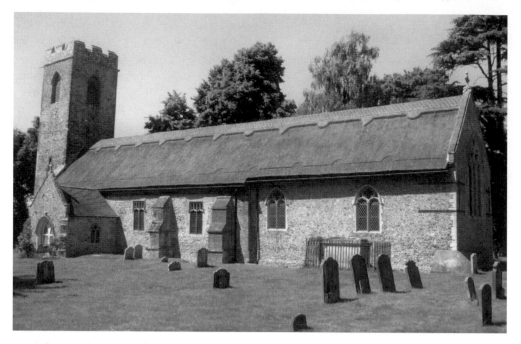

The thatched church at North Cove. (Author's collection)

Realising that something was very wrong indeed, she sent a messenger to find her husband. Matters had worsened by the time Benjamin arrived home, so he immediately set out to walk to Beccles to seek medical assistance. It was noon by the time he reached Beccles and asked Mr Charles Dashwood to attend the family in North Cove. The surgeon agreed that he would call as soon as he could.

It is not known if he offered to take Benjamin back with him in his carriage or left him to make the long journey back on foot. What we do know is that when the surgeon reached the cottage, he found six very pale and shivering children. Questioning those who were old enough to talk, he discovered that they had all experienced stomach cramps. To them he gave the surgeon's standard panacea of an emetic to purge their systems. That Robert was the most seriously ill became obvious when Mr Dashwood, having asked the boy to stand up, found he was far too weak to do so. Realising that prompt action was required, the surgeon ordered a warm bath to be prepared in an attempt to put some heat back into his body. As Robert was gently lowered into the water his stomach muscles contracted and he again convulsed. The little boy died shortly afterwards in Dashwood's arms.

Death coming so rapidly from what had looked at first sight as an outbreak of the usual summer bilious attacks needed further investigation. But before Dashwood added to the distress of the family by performing a post-mortem examination on Robert, he tried to find out what had led up to the sickness. The Sparkes's eldest daughter, a girl of twelve, acted as spokesman. She related how they had all eaten their bread and butter but Robert had been anxious to get on to the cake and taken the first slice and eaten a huge mouthful. The others had followed but when she had bitten into her piece she detected what she described as a bitter taste and, sensing that something was wrong with the cake, she had taken the remains of their slices from each of her brothers and sisters.

The sequence of events following the death is vague. We have to remember that this is the year 1815 and there was news of much greater importance nationally to occupy the local newspaper than the unexplained death of a child in a remote part of Suffolk. Had little Robert Sparkes not been the grandson of his housekeeper, Tifford Clarke himself might not have been concerned with the death. But when he heard that the post-mortem examination on the Tuesday by Dashwood assisted by William Crowfoot, another surgeon from Beccles, had revealed a quantity of arsenic in the remains of the cake in Robert's stomach, he began to wonder. According to one press report, he confided his misgivings to his friend Anthony Fiske, who farmed at Ellingham, asking him to tackle Elizabeth on the subject. She apparently made a full confession to him. Elizabeth was then arrested and brought before the magistrates, Robert Sparrow and John Farr, on Wednesday 5 July, charged with intent to poison Tifford Clarke. She was committed to Beccles Gaol to await trial. There she remained until 17 July when she was taken to Ipswich Gaol in preparation for transfer to Bury St Edmunds, where the Suffolk Summer Assizes were held two days later.

This surely must be one of the speediest cases on record. Less than three weeks after the event Elizabeth was on trial for her life charged with the attempted murder of Tifford Clarke. The case opened at eight o'clock on the morning of Saturday 20 July. Before any evidence was heard, Sir Vicary Gibbs addressed the Grand Jury about the status of case. The jury at an Assize court was drawn from two sources, gentlemen representing the county of Suffolk and those who represented what was then known as a 'Liberty', a smaller administrative area similar to our present-day 'District'. All the members of the jury would have been members of the landowning class and of high standing in their local communities. Gibbs now informed these gentlemen that when the charge had appeared in the Trial Calendar, it was that Elizabeth had mixed a quantity of arsenic in a cake sent to Tifford Clarke with the intention to kill him. However, part of that cake had been eaten by Robert Sparkes which had occasioned his death. But, said Sir Vicary, it did not appear to him that the prisoner was chargeable with any 'malice prepence' (or forethought) against Robert. In other words, Robert's death was an accident.

Evidence was given by the two surgeons of the tests they had carried out to establish the presence of arsenic in the corpse. Then Benjamin Long, a druggist from Bungay, testified that as recently as 22 June, Elizabeth had purchased an ounce of arsenic from him. This was quite a large quantity, but we have to bear in mind that she was a farmer and so her reason for buying – that she wished to control vermin – was perfectly reasonable. So too, according to Vicary, was her reason for buying other amounts three or four times in the past year.

Tifford Clarke was also called and related how Elizabeth had been in the habit of visiting him and bringing gifts, including a cake that had caused him to have an upset stomach. Both Nelson and his fourteen-year-old sister Amy were required to give evidence for the prosecution. Amy, when relating her part in the events, emphasised that her mother had made the cake and that she

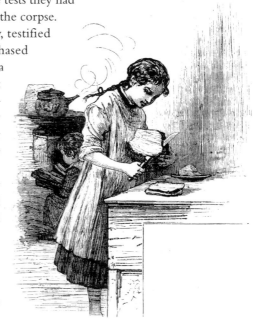

had only packed the basket according to Elizabeth's instructions. The writer of the account of the trial, which appeared in Knapp & Baldwin's Newgate Calendar, described Amy as 'an interesting girl' but failed to elucidate exactly what he meant by that.

Although Elizabeth protested her innocence throughout and despite the plea that she had not intended to kill little Robert, it took the jury just twenty minutes to find her guilty of intent to murder Tifford Clarke and the death penalty was passed upon her.

She was taken back to Ipswich Gaol. Again the execution was to be carried out with great rapidity having been planned for Wednesday 24 July. For some reason it was deferred for a day. Perhaps there had been hope of a reprieve in the form of a commutation of sentence. Unlike later cases, the local newspapers did not give graphic details of the hanging. The *Ipswich Journal* reported simply:

> Thursday last Elizabeth Wooltorton pursuant to her sentence was executed on the drop over the turnkey's lodge of the County gaol for the murder of Robert Sparkes. The unhappy woman was very agitated at the final shot and when asked by Mr Johnson [the gaoler] whether she acknowledged the justice of her sentence she made no intelligible reply and seemed particularly anxious to hide her face from the gaze of the multitude.

The *Suffolk Chronicle* merely noted the execution between a report of a suicide and a coroner's inquest, stating that,

> … the unfortunate woman did not, we understand, make any specific confession of the crime for which she suffered, but admitted in general terms, that she deserved her fate. She appeared to be dreadfully agitated and altogether incapable of supporting herself at the last awful moment.

Although her case had aroused interest, many details were omitted from the press reports in order to give room for the much more important news that Napoleon Bonaparte had finally surrendered and was on his way to Plymouth aboard HMS *Bellerophon*.

When we read these cases, we must wonder what happened afterwards. What, for example, happened to Elizabeth's children, the youngest of whom was only seven years old? We do know that Tifford Clarke lived for another three years. His Will, which runs to some eight pages, shows great generosity towards his housekeeper, Mary Pleasants. He left her the rents from five different properties to provide her with a substantial annuity as well as almost all the contents of his house. He also gave annuities or outright legacies to all her children, including Sarah Sparkes. Six months after young Robert's death, Sarah gave birth to another son, who was also given the name of Robert. He was followed by three more children. Clarke's legacy to them enabled Benjamin to buy his own farm. But perhaps the most interesting of all the legacies was that to Elizabeth's children. In spite of everything, he kept the promise he had made years before to his nephew, and to the Wooltorton children he left each of them a share of the Swan Inn. If only Elizabeth had had a little more patience …

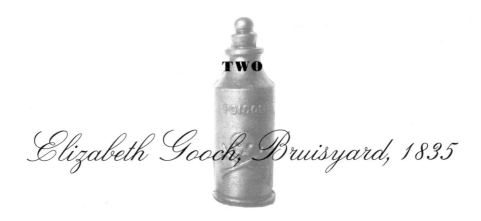

Elizabeth Gooch, Bruisyard, 1835

At around three o'clock on the afternoon of Tuesday, 21 April 1835, Mrs Jane Wells delivered an opened parcel to the house of Mr King, the surgeon in Saxmundham. Used to receiving the occasional gift from grateful patients, George Pretty, King's young apprentice, was no doubt somewhat taken aback when Mrs Wells revealed that inside the wrapping was half a cake – but not for his eating. Instead, she wished Mr King to test it, for she was sure that it contained poison. Pretty, who was on duty alone, took the parcel and left it on the table in the consulting room. Later in the day when Mr Ling, King's assistant, returned from his rounds, he was told the story of the cake and locked it away in a cupboard to await Mr King's return. Ling and Pretty may have discussed the parcel and its contents, possibly dismissing the woman who had brought it as suffering from delusions – otherwise why on earth should she suspect that the gift of a cake was poisoned? After all, according to the addresses on the parcel, it had been sent by her father, Abraham Watson, and, bearing in mind that it had been delivered on the Tuesday after Easter, it could well be a belated gift to her and his two small grandchildren. Jane Wells was a widow and money was short, so the treat of a cake, which must have weighed about a pound, should have been very welcome.

But Jane Wells, who had been widowed two years earlier and lived with her children in the village of Farnham, near from Saxmundham, had strong grounds for believing that the cake contained more than the usual ingredients; for this was not the first unsolicited gift she had received. This time she was determined to get at the truth, so she set out to do her own detective work.

It had been between 8.30 and 9 a.m. on 21 April that Samuel Wainwright, who was employed as a letter-carrier by Mr Keen the Farnham postmaster, had knocked at her door with a parcel. Since carriage was payable by the recipient of the post in those days, Jane, who could not read, asked Wainwright to tell her exactly what was written on the piece of paper held under the string of the parcel just to make sure it really was for her. Told that it said 'Abraham Watson, Thorpe to Jane Wells, Farnham', she handed over the one penny fee and took the parcel in. When she opened it she found five small brown cakes and under them the large cake. Without hesitating, she gave each of the children two of the little cakes and ate the fifth one herself. So what caused her to be so suspicious of the cake that she later divided it up, keeping part and putting the rest back into the wrapper ready to take to Mr King?

Following her afternoon visit to Mr King, Jane made a tour of the cake shops in Saxmundham. Finally, at the home of a Mrs Mills, who sold such items as apples and small

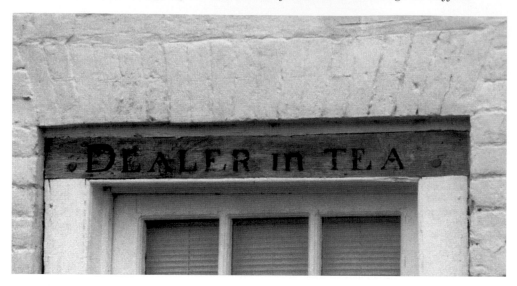

An old shop sign carved over the door of a house in Bruisyard. (Author's collection)

cakes, which she displayed in the window of her cottage, she found the information for which she had been searching. Mrs Mills told her that she had had an early customer at eight o'clock the previous morning. At the time Mrs Mills was busy crumbling bread into milk as breakfast for her five children and so she had not really taken much notice of the woman beyond an overall impression that she had been middle-aged, wearing a light-coloured gown and a black bonnet lined with white. She remembered that she had purchased a pennyworth of brown cakes. She got eight cakes for her penny and these the woman had put into an open parcel she was carrying. As she was leaving she had asked Mrs Mills for directions to the post office.

Jane's next stop was the post office, where she enquired of Mary Stopher, the postmaster's sister and sometime assistant, if she could remember the customer from the previous day who had brought in the parcel. Miss Stopher corroborated the description given by Mrs Mills, adding that the woman had a swarthy complexion, a very prominent nose and high cheekbones. This was sufficient for Jane; she now knew exactly who it was who had sent the parcel, and more importantly, who she suspected had attempted to kill her – and, almost too most horrible to contemplate – her children.

It had to be a woman. Only a woman would have taken the trouble to bake a cake with which to poison another. And if one woman was attempting to kill another, then almost inevitably a man must be involved. And that man was James Maltster, a farm labourer in his thirties. James, who had been born and bred in the village of Bruisyard, near Saxmundham, was a widower with a son and daughter aged eight and six. Since the death of his wife he had had a series of housekeepers to look after them, the latest of which was Elizabeth Gooch, who was also a native of the village. Elizabeth had never married but she had a daughter, Mary, who at sixteen was already married to William Jacobs. Elizabeth supported herself mainly by fieldwork at Bruisyard Hall farm, hence her weather-beaten complexion. When outside work was not available she was employed in the farmhouse where, among other duties, she did all the laundry. John Baldry, the farm foreman who had known her for almost nine years, reckoned her to be a most conscientious and trustworthy worker. He had never seen any sign

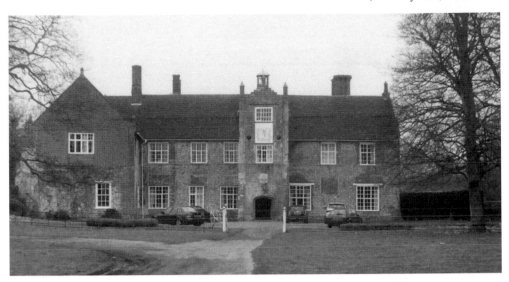

Bruisyard Hall, where Elizabeth Gooch was employed. (Author's collection)

of malice or ill temper in either her speech or actions so he had taken her word for it that she really was troubled with mice, when, in the previous November, she had asked for a bit of arsenic. He had let her have about a tablespoonful from the store he kept for steeping his wheat seeds in before they were sown.

In 1835, Elizabeth was about forty-five. In an age when a large proportion of the rural population was illiterate and the passage of time was marked by the seasons, the actual number of the year was irrelevant even if known. So it is not always possible to give someone an accurate age, because people were often unsure of when they had been born. For the years before birth certificates were issued, researchers have to rely on the Church's records for a date of a child's baptism. Although this event was supposed to take place within a few weeks of a child's birth, there were often reasons why this did not happen. Clergymen in small parishes often held baptismal services only two or three times a year, so the baby might have been born in the year previous to the one in the register. And sometimes, perhaps because the parents had moved several times, all the children in the family were baptised *en bloc*, but the register would give no indication how old each was. Few were the clergy who insisted on accuracy and gave a birth date for the child as well as a baptismal one, thus establishing an exact age. When the census was taken in 1851 the enumerators had either to take the word of the householder or make a shrewd guess as to age. This explains why, when following a subject through the various census years, there may be discrepancies.

Like the majority of villages at that time, most of the inhabitants of Bruisyard, if not directly related, knew each other. So it was that James had known Elizabeth for much of his life. But she had only moved into his home at the end of the previous September, on Michaelmas Day, the traditional day for rural employment contracts to begin and end. It seems that the post of housekeeper carried with it the tacit understanding that the woman would share the bed of her employer. This may initially have been a matter of necessity, the employer's bed being the only one with any room in it. Sharing beds was not considered unusual in the early nineteenth century, even in wealthier households than those we are dealing with here; maids would sleep with their mistresses on occasion, and male travellers might well be expected to share a bed with a total stranger in a wayside inn.

The 'honeymoon period' had lasted about three or four months and then the arguments began. James accused Elizabeth of using bad language and Elizabeth, perhaps being kept short of housekeeping money, accused James of starving his children. But the truth of the situation was that James had grown tired of the older woman who, whatever other qualities she possessed, could not be called a beauty, and his eye had been caught by the younger and more attractive Jane Wells. Since Jane, Elizabeth and James had all known each other for at least eight years, we must assume that she too had lived in Bruisyard at some time, perhaps moving to Farnham following her husband's death. Whatever the circumstances, Jane and James had renewed their earlier acquaintance sometime at the end of February and soon he was making regular evening visits to Farnham as their friendship deepened.

James made no secret of where he now often spent the evening, leaving Elizabeth alone in the house with his children. More quarrels followed. In one, Elizabeth threatened that if James ever brought Jane into the house she would do her a mischief. Returning one evening he reputedly said, 'Well, Mrs Gooch, you're home from your washing,' to which she replied, 'And well, Mr Maltster, you are got home from your whore.' Things became worse between them. Throughout March, James spent more and more time at Farnham, often returning in a belligerent mood. Elizabeth had grown fearful of his temper so she asked her daughter Mary to come and stay. The two were in bed when James came in at around two in the morning. He thundered into the bedroom, got hold of the bedcovers and threw them down the narrow twisting staircase at the edge of the room and then made a lunge at the bed, which broke. Wildly he grabbed at Mary, holding her tightly round the waist, preparing to throw her after the bedclothes, yelling, 'I'll hurl you downstairs and if I kill you I don't mind being hung for you.' The tension of the situation eased somewhat when he discovered that it was Mary in his grasp and not Elizabeth.

In spite of everything, Elizabeth was determined not to lose him so she made the journey to Farnham, where she angrily confronted Jane about the relationship and warned her she must have nothing more to do with him – or else! Although Elizabeth warned Jane she was to say nothing to James about her visit, she did, of course. After that, he must have decided he could no longer bear to be in the same house as Elizabeth, so on 25 March he left. The parting was acrimonious, with a scuffle taking place in the street outside the cottage as Elizabeth tried to prevent him from going. It ended with James knocking her to the ground and leaving her lying in the road kicking and screaming in a hysterical fit. What is not clear is why he left the house rather than simply sacking her and sending her away. He, after all, was the tenant of the cottage. Neither is there any indication of what happened to his children. We are forced therefore to assume that it was for their sake that he vacated the house because he still expected Elizabeth to look after them. Quite where he went is also uncertain, as Jane was later to swear in court that he was not living with her.

Elizabeth was inconsolable once he had gone and Mary, who had now been joined by her husband in the house, began to fear for her mother's sanity. For two or three days and nights she not only cried but she also raved wildly, convinced that people were coming to take her away. Scarily for Mary, the two men who were to do this, whom Elizabeth named as Mr Hart of Cranfield and Mr Hanton of Bruisyard, were both dead!

Once her tears had subsided, Elizabeth began to plan her revenge. At the beginning of April she sent two bottles to Jane. The account of this story in the *Suffolk Chronicle* does not state what these two bottles contained but it would most likely have been home-brewed beer. Alternatively, the *Ipswich Journal* reported that she sent Jane two letters. The former is the more likely and even more likely was Jane's fear that the contents of the bottles contained poison. James had no doubt told her that Elizabeth had arsenic in the house to deal with mice. If it was indeed two bottles that were sent, then presumably Elizabeth expected the couple would drink from them and so she would dispose of them both. Bottles or letters, it does not matter which because when delivered to her door, Jane refused to accept them. No doubt she told James what had occurred and it may be that he then added fuel to the fire of suspicion by suggesting that he had seen Elizabeth mixing arsenic with flour. Hence her firm belief that the cake, when it arrived, was poisoned.

A week or so after taking the cake to Mr King, Jane had heard nothing, so she took the other piece to him. It appears that the original piece was still locked in the cupboard in the surgery! Presented with the other half, Mr King was galvanised into action. He immediately dispatched one piece to London for detailed analysis and the other he took to his own laboratory in Aldeburgh, where he carried out his experiments. Both he and his London colleague applied a number of tests and both achieved the same result of metallic arsenic. There was no doubt that the cake was impregnated with sufficient arsenic to cause death. Eating just a normal slice would have proved lethal if prompt medical treatment was not given.

Elizabeth was promptly arrested by a young police constable, Edward Kell of Bruisyard, who had the task of keeping her in his custody for several days until her appearance before the magistrates in Framlingham, where she was charged with attempted murder. They believed the evidence presented to them was sufficient for her to be sent for trial at the Summer Assizes in Bury St Edmunds, held at the end of July. It would appear that this early triumph encouraged PC Kell in his career, for we find him later holding the rank of sergeant in the London borough of Hornsey.

Among the witnesses called to appear for the prosecution were Mrs Mills and Miss Stopher. Mrs Mills had recently given birth to her sixth child and there was some doubt as to her state of health and whether she would be fit enough to make the journey to Bury. (*See* Appendix - Mr Clubbe's Accounts.) Both women testified that they had identified Elizabeth at Framlingham but each made the point that the prisoner they now saw at the bar was considerably thinner than the one they had seen that April day in Saxmundham. Indeed much emphasis was laid on the prisoner's appearance. The reporter of the *Suffolk Chronicle* wrote that she was not at all prepossessing, using the words 'cadaverous' and 'wrinkled'. The description of her prominent nose and exceptionally high cheekbones, accentuated by her loss of weight, conjures up an image of the storybook witch. The reporter also suggested that Elizabeth appeared to be in the last stages of mental wretchedness.

An important but reluctant witness was eighteen-year-old John Fisk of Bruisyard, an agricultural labourer who occasionally worked with James Maltster. Like everyone else in the village, Fisk knew that 'old Betty', as he called her, was living with Maltster as his housekeeper. He thought it was either on Easter Sunday, or possibly the Sunday before, that she had asked him to do her a favour. She wanted to send two letters but as she could not write, she was going to get someone who could to do it for her. However, that person could not write names, so she asked him to write the names and addresses for her. As she dictated he wrote on two separate pieces of paper 'Abraham Watson, Thorpe and Jane Wells, Farnham.' Fisk identified his handwriting on the paper attached to the parcel but denied that he had ever discussed Elizabeth with James.

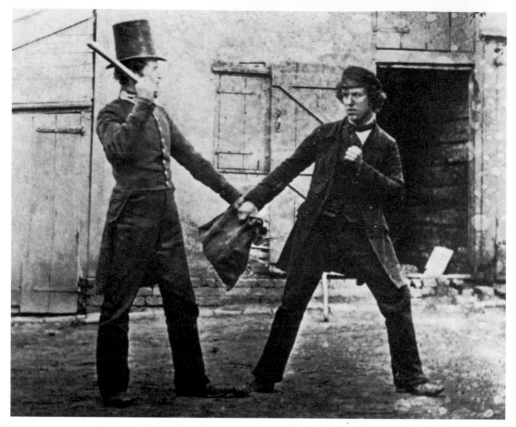

Police uniform of the period. (Robert Burrows. Reproduced by kind permission of SRO/ Ipswich)

The trial had its lighter moments. At one point after Jane had described the cake as having been cooked in a tin, the judge demanded to know if James had such cake tins in his house and, having been told that he had, then wanted to know why the tin had not been produced in court. Later on, while James was giving his evidence, Elizabeth challenged him. She addressed the judge, saying, 'I hope your Lordship will be pleased to hear me after you have heard his story.' Unfortunately we are not told of his Lordship's response to this. However, he seems to have ignored this outburst as well as what amounted to a slanging match between the pair across the courtroom. Elizabeth managed to get in her reference to his whore before she collapsed in a fit. She was removed from the court for a short while only to be brought back in what appeared to be an inanimate state, so she was taken out again. Fortunately Mr King, the surgeon, was still present so he attended to her. When she was able to return to the dock, Mr King told the court that she was not epileptic, but that she was suffering from a real illness caused by the excitement of the trial.

The defence lawyer used this event to concentrate on Elizabeth's mental state. Another witness, John Smith of Bruisyard, testified he had known her all her life and had never seen any sign of malice in her. However, on the night of Easter Monday, when he saw her in the local inn, he had noted that she looked like 'a wild woman'. James had been present in the inn too but as far as Smith knew they had not spoken to each other. However, he did admit that it was common knowledge in the village that there was a dispute between the two.

The last witness for the defence was Mary Jacob. She told the court of James's abusive behaviour to her mother and gave a graphic account of the night he had grabbed her out of the bed. She had been frightened then for herself as well as for her mother. She also told of the deep mental anguish Elizabeth had suffered after James left the house. When she gave the account of Elizabeth's fears of being taken away, there was a sudden shriek from the prisoner. Yet again Elizabeth was removed from the courtroom.

The case concluded and the jury retired. When they returned the foreman handed the judge a written verdict that,

> ... at the time of committing the offence, the jury considered the prisoner to be in such a state of insane mind as not to be able to distinguish right from wrong being under the influence of strongly irritated feelings; they begged to accompany a verdict of Guilty with a strong recommendation of mercy.

This, as it stood, was not acceptable in the eyes of the law and the judge went to some lengths to explain various points. As it stood, Elizabeth was accused of attempted murder. The evidence against her was strong. If they found her guilty then the sentence must be death. There was, however, one loophole and the judge offered it to them.

Judge: 'A verdict for acquittal must be satisfied that when she mixed the poison she did not know right from wrong.'
Foreman: 'We believe she was in an irritable state of mind as not to be actually cognisant at all times of her actions.'
Judge: 'In order to acquit her you must find her insane. I can receive this verdict in the form you have given but it would not amount to an acquittal on the grounds of insanity.'
Foreman: 'The jury do not mean to acquit her on the ground of insanity.'
Judge: 'Then you simply recommend mercy on account of a disordered state of mind?'
Foreman: 'Yes.'
Judge: 'Then I receive the verdict and I shall take note of your recommendation.'

The judge then ordered that the prisoner should be brought back the next day for sentencing.

We may question why the jury did not take the offer of the plea of insanity. Was it that they did not regard being held in a lunatic asylum as sufficient punishment, or was it simply that they admitted her guilt and were asking for the death penalty to be commuted? There is no way of knowing. What we do know is that Elizabeth Gould was sentenced to death even though no one was actually poisoned. However, mercy was shown and her sentence was commuted to transportation for life.

Within three months, Elizabeth was placed on board the convict ship the *Henry Wellesley*, which sailed from Portsmouth on 7 October bound for New South Wales. After a journey of 123 days the ship reached its destination on 7 February 1836.

As for James Maltster, he did not marry Jane Wells. Perhaps the relationship could not stand the strain of being in the public eye. In July 1841 a James Maltster, widower of Bruisyard, married the widow Sarah Mowson. If this is our James, then it is interesting that Sarah's occupation, like that of Elizabeth, was given as washerwoman. It also appears that James had a preference for older women, as his new wife was some seven years his senior.

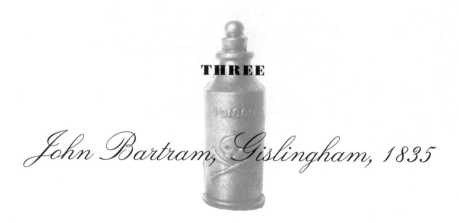

THREE

John Bartram, Gislingham, 1835

Not all deaths from arsenic were the result of deliberate murder, but even where this was the case it was rare that more than one or two people were involved, so the headline in the *Ipswich Journal* of 22 August 1835 of 'Twenty-three persons poisoned at Gislingham in Suffolk' must surely have grabbed the readers' attention. Those who might have feared that a mass murderer was on the loose in this village five miles south west of the market town of Eye, must then have been reassured to learn this massive outbreak of poisoning was in fact caused by eating bread made from contaminated flour. Furthermore, it had been confined to the members of four large families, all of whom had been taken so seriously ill that two of them had died.

The awful events revolved around the family of Jacob Taylor. Jacob was an agricultural labourer. He was thirty-seven years old, in good health and well thought of by both his employer and his neighbours. He and his wife had five children ranging in age from fourteen to a baby of six months. Within their very limited means, Mrs Taylor did her best to keep their cottage home neat and clean and the family decently clothed and fed. However, they, and many like them, had suffered difficulties in recent months, and as a result had had to call on Parish Relief. They had needed both a ration of coal and money to get them through the winter and early spring. Perhaps it was to add a few extra pence to their income that they had taken in a lodger. John Bartram was also receiving benefit from the Poor Rate. In his case the Overseers had been making regular weekly payments for his lodging and for his being 'in need' for some time. His need was such that on 29 September 1834 the sum of 1s 9d was paid out to provide him with a pair of stockings. Bartram had a bed in the house but not board, that is, he did not eat with the family but provided his own food.

Mrs Taylor was in the habit of buying her flour in bulk from Mr Wright, the baker from nearby Finningham. About three weeks before they were all taken ill, she had received 140lbs of flour, about half a sack, from Mr Wright, who had delivered it to her door and then carried it through to the pantry for her. While it was there she had used some of it to make her usual batch of bread. Then the sack was moved to what was described as a ground-floor bedroom, where John Bartram slept. There is no indication of how big the room was.

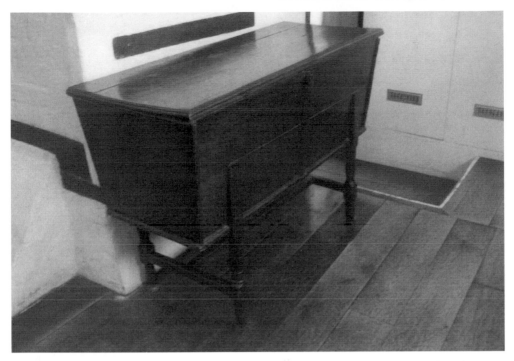

A kneading trough, Christchurch Mansion, Ipswich. (Author's collection)

We know only that its walls were white-washed, probably like the rest of the interior of the cottage, and that there was a high shelf along one wall where shoes were kept. Most cottages at that period consisted of a kitchen/living room and some had a small room leading off it which was used for many different purposes.

Just before Jacob left for work at 6 a.m. on Thursday 5 August, Mrs Taylor asked if he would 'shoot' part of the flour from the sack into her flour trough. He emptied out about three stones and then returned the sack to the back room. As soon as Jacob left, Mrs Taylor got down to work making a number of loaves of bread, some puddings and 'sweet cakes', probably similar to fruit scone rounds. Her output was considerable as she used about three quarters of the flour, four pounds of flour being used in each quartern loaf of bread. By seven o'clock the bread mixture was ready to be left to rise at the end of the trough opposite to the remaining flour. The loaves and cakes were put into the oven at about eleven o'clock and for supper that night the family sat down to freshly baked bread. Jacob, having spent the day in the fields, took one of his wife's sweet cakes with him when he went to the Six Bells public house later that night.

Like most nursing mothers at that time, Mrs Taylor was supplementing the baby's feed with what was commonly known as 'pap' – bread soaked in milk. Within ten minutes or so of the baby being fed, she brought it all back. This did not cause too much worry but then Charlotte, who was two and a half, vomited too, followed shortly afterwards by John, the eldest child, and finally the other two.

Jacob had a slice of bread for his breakfast the next morning but the children, still upset from the night before, did not. At that stage, bread would have been the last thing suspected of causing a stomach upset. Certainly Mrs Taylor had not hesitated to lend two of her loaves to a neighbour, Mrs Osborn, who had run out of bread and had seven hungry children to feed. Feeling better by Saturday morning, the Taylors had their usual breakfast of bread and butter but were soon retching and vomiting throughout the day – so much so that Jacob begged a ride in a cart for the four-mile journey to Rickinghall to seek the advice of Mr Vincent. The surgeon's opinion was that Jacob was probably suffering from a fever brought on by the heat, and the vomiting was the result of drinking newly brewed beer. Harvest time involved extra long hours in the fields exposed to the sun and the very nature of reaping and stacking the corn was known to be very thirsty work. Thus Mr Vincent prescribed emetics for the whole family.

Early on Sunday morning John Bartram was also sick. When, later in the day, Mrs Taylor got Jacob to offer him some of her bread because he had not eaten all day, he refused it and told her, 'if you eat that bread you will all certainly be poisoned.' He said it seemed 'sour'. No doubt Mrs Taylor took this as a slight on her cooking. And in any case by this time the rest of the family seemed to have recovered and not be in need of the dose of emetics brought to them by the doctor's apprentice. Being Sunday, the Taylors had visitors, Jacob's widowed sister-in-law and her two children and another nephew called John Pitcher. In the afternoon they all sat down to a dinner, at which was served one of the puddings Mrs Taylor had made earlier. Shortly after they had finished they all showed signs of either feeling very unwell or actually vomiting. The guests decided to cut short their visit and go home.

John Bartram was out of the house for most of that day but he did make an unexpected call on Thomas Talbot. Telling about the situation in the Taylor household, Bartram asked if Talbot would give him some bread and cakes for the children. Talbot gave him some and when Bartram had gone he found, much to his surprise, that he had left sixpence in payment. Later that evening, Mrs Taylor had just gone upstairs to bed with Jacob preparing to follow her when their lodger arrived home the worse for drink. In his drunken ravings he begged Jacob to dispose of their bread, saying, 'Taylor boy, if you eat that bread you will surely be poisoned.' Believing this was the beer talking, Jacob went upstairs but before he had time to get into bed, Bartram called him down again and repeated the warning. Trying once again to get to his bed, Jacob remarked to his wife, 'Good God, what has he got into his head, he fare wholly crazy.' Bartram then begged both of them to come down, which they did, no doubt very reluctantly, only to find him lying across the foot of his bed, trembling all over as if either in a fever or a fit. In his ranting he begged Mrs Taylor not to eat the bread and allegedly said to them, 'I'll be damned if I'm not dying.'

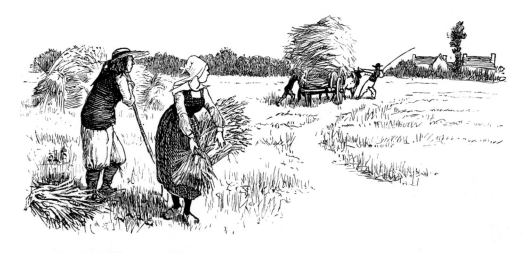

After their disturbed night, Jacob was up early to leave for work at six o'clock as usual. He had a bit of bread and butter before he left but it was not long before he was taken so ill in the fields that he was sent home. He had not been there long when the woman who lived in the adjacent cottage called to tell Mrs Taylor that all nine of the Osborn family were just as sick as the Taylors were since they had eaten her bread. Jacob lost his temper somewhat at this imputation and strode off to the Osborns, where he ended up buying a peck (a bucketful) of potatoes. Although Jacob was feeling queasy, he was not as ill as Mrs Taylor had now become so he boiled some of the potatoes to feed the rest of the family. Jacob and young Charlotte both ate bread with their potatoes while the others just had potatoes. For some reason Jacob could not sit still to eat but paced round the room. Sometime later, between six and seven o'clock, he was seized with such violent pain that he was convinced he was dying. He must also have felt in need of fresh air for he went out into the back yard and sat on a bank, where he retched. While he was suffering outside the house, little Charlotte was inside enduring similar symptoms. It was then that Jacob decided to consign the rest of the bread to the swill bucket.

He managed to get to work the next day but returned in the evening feeling very unwell. On his way he called in at one of the local shops where William Garrard, the owner, advised him not to eat any more of the family bread. It was good advice, but as bread was the staple diet of the time, to buy it put an additional strain on the family budget. On Wednesday, Jacob again struggled to work. Time off work meant less in his pay at the end of the week but on that day he was so weak he was brought home in one of the farm wagons. He went straight to his bed, unable to help Charlotte, who died that day. The following day, still very weak, he hitched a lift in the grocer's cart to see Mr Vincent. Then he returned home to bed.

Meanwhile, at the Six Bells on that Thursday, the local magistrate, Charles Gross, held the inquest into the sudden death of Charlotte. It was at best a rather brief affair and what evidence was given was not properly recorded. The verdict was 'death occasioned by arsenic mixed with bread but how or by what means it became mixed, no evidence appeared to the jury.' It is to be presumed that since Mrs Taylor was as ill as the rest of the family, there was no hint of suggestion that she as the maker of the bread had been responsible for her daughter's death.

As he lay in his sickbed that day, Jacob must have turned over and over in his fevered brain the question of poison and how it had got into the bread. The horror of one of the possibilities may account for the conversation he had with a Mary Barton, who called to see how he was. During their conversation, Jacob reputedly said of the poisoning 'no man did this', to which Mary had retorted, 'it must be a woman then. Have you suspicions?' Jacob had replied, 'yes I have, but I'll never say.' Mary of course drew the obvious conclusion that Jacob was pointing the finger at his wife. Whether he really believed that we shall never know and he certainly did not mention it when later that same day he asked Thomas Talbot to visit him. Talbot was a man of strong religious faith. A member of the chapel he may also have been a lay-preacher. It was to Talbot that John Bartram had gone the previous Sunday for bread and cakes for the Taylor children but Jacob needed Talbot's spiritual comfort. The death of his daughter may have made him realise that he was unlikely to recover his own health. So asking Talbot to read from the Bible, he requested Psalm 103, very much a prayer for a life nearing its end, one certain of forgiveness for past sins and the enduring love and mercy of the Lord. Jacob was making his peace with his maker. Before Talbot left, Jacob asked to pray with him.

After leaving the house, Talbot met Bartram in the street. He stopped to speak, commenting on the sad news of the death of one of the Taylor children. To Talbot's surprise Bartram said that it was good news as it meant Taylor would have one less mouth to feed. He went on to say that it would be even better if two or three more children were to be taken. He then remarked, 'Damn it, if that they had money, there would be nobody die, if life could be bought with money.' Leaving Talbot to work out exactly what he meant, Bartram went on his way.

Meanwhile, Mrs Taylor, herself very weak, was coping with the death of one child and the sickness of the rest of them. John, the eldest, had now added severe pains in his head to his symptoms and then, at about seven o'clock on Friday morning, Jacob suffered a nosebleed that nothing would staunch. Mr Vincent was called and found when he arrived at 11 a.m. that Jacob was still haemorrhaging. He managed to stem the flow but by that time Jacob was very weak.

His condition worsened overnight much to the concern of Rebecca Rocket, a villager who was acting as night nurse. At four o'clock on Saturday morning she decided to send again for the surgeon. Mrs Taylor set out to ask Mr Garrard, who had transport, if he would go for Mr Vincent. John Bartram, hearing movements, got up and said he would go with her. When they reached Mr Garrard's gate, she was going to leave Bartram and go in on her own but Bartram begged her not to leave him. 'Pray Mistress, don't leave me for I durst not be alone – they will certainly shoot us.' He then asked repeatedly, 'Where shall I go to – sure Taylor won't die.' When Mrs Taylor said she feared that he was already dying, the man would not have it.

Mr Vincent eventually came and this time diagnosed that Jacob had inflammation of the lungs. By then he had the evidence from Charlotte's inquest so he was pretty safe in assuming that Jacob was also suffering from arsenic poisoning. When Mr Vincent questioned him, he recalled they had had arsenic in the house some three years previously but having children around he had been very careful to make sure that when he put it into the mouse holes, they had been immediately filled in. The dying man was by now convinced that John Bartram was responsible for poisoning the flour.

Jacob lasted another fourteen hours, dying around six o'clock on Saturday evening, and in the early hours of Sunday, a neighbour, Dinah Seaman, laid out his corpse. When Bartram heard the news he asked to speak to Mrs Taylor. She was busy making tea for her female helpers and told him he would have to wait. Eventually, he could stand it no longer and demanded her attention. He confessed that he had brought some poison into the house about six weeks earlier. For safekeeping he had stowed it inside an old shoe that stood on the shelf above the flour sack. One day he had reached up to get his highlows (a type of boot) ready to go into the fields to do some reaping and as he did so he had knocked down the shoe that held the poison. As it fell its contents were scattered on the sack below. He had panicked and had tried to scoop it out, putting the top layer of flour into a bag he had found in one of Mrs Taylor's drawers. But then, overcome with fear, he had thrown the bag back into the flour trough. When Mrs Taylor asked him why he hadn't told her, he said he had been too frightened. Having got his confession off his chest he then asked where Jacob was. When she said he was dead he did not believe her so she took him up to view the corpse. At the sight of it Bartram appeared, in Mrs Taylor's words, 'quite struck and quite in a stupid state for a minute or two.' Then he went downstairs, out of the house and ran away through the hedge, apparently in a deranged state.

What happened next is not clear but at some stage Bartram was taken into custody by the Gislingham constable and held overnight on Sunday ready for the inquest on Jacob on Monday. In his statement to the police, Bartram now told a different story to the one he had related to Mrs Taylor. In this version it was the young Osborn boys who had thrown arsenic powder all over his clothes while he had been in their barn. Or they might have put some in his pockets without his knowing. However it had got there, one night when he took off his waistcoat and flung it on top of the flour sack it had fallen out and that was how the flour was contaminated.

The inquest on Jacob was held on Monday 17 August. The jury was composed of seventeen men and also present were Sir Augustus Henniker and the Revd Thomas Collyer. Their first duty was to view the body still lying in the Taylors' home. On entering the cottage they were greeted by the piteous sight of the still very weak widow propped up in a chair, a kindly neighbour was helping to nurse a very sick seven-year-old-girl, while lying in its cradle was the equally ailing baby and in a makeshift bed lay young John, apparently close to death. Upstairs they found Jacob, 'a most ghastly corpse', shrouded in his coffin.

By the time Bartram was brought before the inquest on Monday, although he was able to repeat the oath, he gave the impression that he had lost his sanity. Mr Gross, the magistrate, asked him if he remembered the day before, to which Bartram replied twice that he did remember one day. When asked if he knew where poor Taylor was, he expressed the hope that he was in heaven; he didn't know but he hoped he was. Pressed on the matter of the arsenic he agreed that he had some that he had got from Mr Garrard. This suggested that he had bought it from the shop, but according to Bartram he had found some in the fields belonging to Mr Garrard, where it was being used for steeping wheat. Yes, he had taken some, in fact he now remembered he had stolen it. This fitted the account Bartram had given Thomas Talbot when he told him he had never bought poison but he did have some. Talbot said he had known Bartram for nearly twenty years; there was no malice in him, he was simply half-witted. That he was not malicious is questionable, for when he was asked about the bag belonging to Mrs Taylor that had been found hidden, he said Mrs Taylor had told him it contained poisoned flour. As for the poison that was supposed to have been in the shoe, Bartram now said he believed Mrs Taylor must have put it there. The coroner took the unusual step of offering Bartram a slice of bread. The man took it and even though he was told it was poisoned, he bit into it. Having tasted it he announced that it was nasty. He then said, 'I know what will hurt – yes I do. I tasted of the arsenic at Osborn's barn. The boys tried to take it away but I only put enough on my fingers to taste it. I know what would hurt me.'

The inquest lasted ten hours. During his summing up, Mr Gross took Mr Vincent to task for his medical treatment of the poor. He suggested that his simply doling out magnesia powders and ordering them to drink milk hardly amounted to careful diagnosis. He indirectly reminded Vincent that while the poor did not pay as well as his rich patients, as a Poor Law doctor he was paid a regular income to take care of them. The inquest verdict was similar to that which had been passed on Charlotte, namely that death was the result of arsenic in the bread. John Bartram was declared not sane and therefore not responsible for his actions and an order was made for his immediate transfer to Melton Union House, which specialised in the care of the mentally ill.

This was an unexpected verdict. Bartram had confessed to being in possession of the poison; it then being introduced into the flour, albeit accidentally, the coroner might well have suggested that he had a case to answer in court, especially as he had caused two deaths with the likelihood that there might be more. There was hardly any mention of police involvement in the case either. One wonders how mentally ill Bartram really was. The villagers had for years recognised that he was, in their words, 'half-witted' and tolerated his behaviour, but now they realised he was a danger. Did the presence of the local landowner Lord Henniker at the inquest have any significance? Did he and the vicar feel that no real purpose would be served by bringing Bartram to trial? Although ordered to Melton Asylum, this in itself was not necessarily a life sentence. His maintenance costs there would be borne by the parish and if he showed signs of improvement or being cured then he would be released. Certainly he fared much better than most of the others in this book.

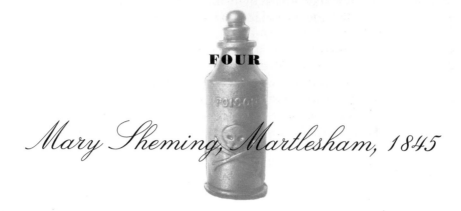

FOUR

Mary Sheming, Martlesham, 1845

Of all forms of murder, the killing of a child generates the strongest abhorrent reaction from the public. It is bad enough when the killer is unknown, but when an innocent life is taken by a member of his or her own family, nothing but anger, hatred and revulsion is directed at the perpetrator. In Suffolk all these emotions were built up to fever pitch when Mary Sheming was brought to trial accused of the murder of her baby grandson.

The Shemings lived in Martlesham, a village close to Ipswich on the road to Woodbridge. Thomas, who was coming up to sixty, was an agricultural labourer who had done his best over the years to support his family. By 1844 he was hoping that at least one of his two sons and three of the four daughters, who ranged in age from twenty-four to eleven, might help contribute to the family finances so that he would not be forced to seek Parish Relief, as he had some ten years earlier. The girls still lived at home but went out daily to do domestic work. They were not allowed to live-in at their place of employment after the eldest girl, sixteen-year-old Caroline, became pregnant by a local farmer and had to return home, where she had remained with her baby daughter, Elizabeth, thus giving poor Thomas another two mouths to feed.

When Caroline was able to work again, she left her mother to look after the infant. In her forties and with her own youngest child within a year or two of being able to work, Mary probably did not relish having to start baby rearing all over again. Caroline seems to have been a somewhat feckless mother and within a year or so she took herself off to Lowestoft, leaving little Elizabeth with her grandparents. Whether this move was to find work or because she accompanied a man there, is not known. Given the proximity of Martlesham to Waldringfield, it is possible that she had met a sailor or fisherman there who encouraged her to join him in his home port. What is known is that in the early part of 1844 she realised she was pregnant again. Her son, John, was born in Lowestoft 'three days before Whitsun', that is about 7 May. Three or four weeks later, she turned up at her parents' house expecting to be taken in. Since Caroline was without money, we are left to assume that she either did not know who the father was or that the man in question had refused to admit his paternity. The Poor Law Overseers, who were asked to approve the provision of financial support from the Parish Poor Rate for illegitimate children, were quick to pursue putative fathers with bastardy orders, which meant regular payments were collected from them either weekly or, in the case of gentlemen of means, by the investment of a lump sum.

As happened so often in the summer months, sickness was rife and both of Caroline's children were ill during the latter part of July. In fact Mary was deeply concerned about the now three-year-old Elizabeth. On the Sunday before the alleged murder took place she was in her garden when Henry Jay, the local wheelwright, stopped for a chat. Part of Henry's work was to make coffins for the villagers and Mary confided to him that he might soon have another order, for her little granddaughter was very poorly. During their conversation she confided that her daughter had received no maintenance from the father of the second child and that unless Caroline could get Parish Relief there would be nothing else for it but for her to take the children into the Union House of Industry – the local workhouse. Thomas Sheming could no longer continue to support the children without some assistance.

The baby had developed a cold as well as thrush. Both conditions had made him very fretful for several days; so much so that Mary demanded that Caroline must look after the child herself, to let her get on with her own work. She had no time to sit and nurse an irritable child for hours on end, in fact, for the three or four days prior to Tuesday 30 July, she had very little to do with him, neither feeding him or picking him up. However, on that day she heard that she had a letter awaiting collection at the post office in Woodbridge so she asked Caroline to go and fetch it for her in the early evening. Although the baby was not yet three months old, Caroline was supplementing breast milk with pap or sop – finely crumbled bread soaked in milk. Some had been given to the baby at noon, with the rest of the mixture put in a cupboard for use later. Before she left at six o'clock, Caroline suckled the infant then told her mother to give him the pap should he appear to be hungry.

After she had had gone the baby did not settle to sleep, which annoyed Mary, as she wanted to finish brewing her beer. So she left Elizabeth to nurse him while she busied herself in the brew-house. Young as she was, Elizabeth had become accustomed to looking after the baby. She managed to get him to sleep for a bit but when Mary had finished her tasks, she came back to the kitchen to find the baby screaming. She immediately took the child and, believing him to be hungry, instructed Elizabeth to fetch the bowl of pap and warm it by the fire. Mary then stirred some milk and butter into the mixture, warning the little girl to make sure it was not too hot. While she was feeding him the baby's eyes suddenly started to roll. Frightened, Mary gave him back to Elizabeth to hold while she went for help.

It was sometime between eight and nine o'clock that she ran across to her neighbour, Mrs Brett, to ask her to come and look at the child. When Mrs Brett went into the Shemings' house, where she found Elizabeth with the baby in her lap, the first thing she saw was that the baby had been sick. The elderly Mrs Brett opined that she didn't like the look of the baby at all. She said so again a few minutes later when Caroline returned, adding brusquely that she was surprised she had gone out leaving her child in such a state. Caroline replied tartly that he had been perfectly all right when she left. She then turned on her mother and asked what she had given him. Mary assured her that he had had nothing but the sop. Mrs Brett then recommended they should give the baby that panacea of all ills, an emetic. According to Mrs Brett's later testimony, Mary had scoffed at this, saying, 'an emetic won't do any good, for it won't be here but a very few hours.' Mrs Brett, who we are to assume had witnessed sickness and death amongst many of her neighbours during her long life, assured them she could not see any sign of imminent death in the child. Her advice was that Caroline should take him into bed with her and keep a rush light burning so that she could keep an eye on him during the night.

Mrs Brett returned home to bed. Within an hour Mary called her to come again as the baby was a great deal worse. By the time Mrs Brett arrived she found Mary was preparing to go to her bed, which was in a corner of the living room, so she was directed to the bedroom, where she found Caroline in bed with the baby. The baby was in such a distressed state that Mrs Brett instinctively picked him up in an attempt to pacify him. Sensing the seriousness of the situation, she told Caroline to get up and call her mother. Mrs Brett continued to try and soothe the child but he strained against her as if racked by excruciating pain. Three hours later there was a sudden gush of foam from the baby's mouth, which, Mrs Brett noticed, contained some 'white stuff'. For her this was proof that had the baby been given the emetic she had recommended earlier he would have been purged that much quicker. However, it was too late. Baby John died around two o'clock in the morning. Mrs Brett did what was necessary and then went home.

She returned at around eight o'clock that morning and looked carefully at the baby, as if seeking for signs that would explain his death. What she could not understand was why Mary seemed so reluctant to touch the tiny corpse. Having been asked to come and put clean clothes on the baby prior to his burial, when she sought Mary's assistance to hold the baby's head, the grandmother recoiled from the task. Caroline was similarly unable to help, being apparently overcome with grief. So it was left to Mrs Brett to help Henry Jay place the child in its tiny coffin.

It may seem odd that Thomas Sheming seems to have played no part at all in any of the events surrounding the death of his grandson. It was Mrs Brett who later related that Thomas, being worn out after having worked all day in the harvest fields, had come home and gone to bed. One imagines that he regarded the sickness of children as women's work and so of little concern to him. Possibly he slept throughout all the events of the evening. Thus it was left to Mary to deal with the formalities. First there was the visit to Robert Smy, the Registrar and Relieving Officer of Colneis District, to register little John's death. She gave the cause of death as convulsion. At this point in our investigation of this case we come across an anomaly that seems to have passed with little comment at the time. All the evidence was that John had died on 30 July, yet according to each of the three newspapers, which carried accounts, Robert Smy testified at the inquest on John that he was asked for a death certificate on 19 July for a child who had died of convulsions on the 13th of that month. A copy of John's death certificate shows that he died at 2 a.m. on 13 July 1844 and was registered by Mary on 19 July. The registrar named in the newspaper accounts as Smy was actually called Thomas Miles. When asked in court about the date of the registration of the death, he admitted that he was very busy attending to paupers at the time and he had written the date of the nineteenth. The certificate also states that the child was three weeks old, not months, and perhaps even more careless on Mr Miles's part, he had first written the word 'daughter' instead of 'son'. It was an error that was immediately corrected. However, this is a salutary reminder that even legal documents from the past may be incorrect.

Once she had the death certificate, Mary visited Mr Pawson, the minister of Waldringfield Baptist Church, to arrange for the burial in the graveyard there. This is the only occasion among the burials described in this book where the victim was interred anywhere other than the graveyard of the parish church according to the rites of the Church of England. It is possible that the Sheming family were Non-conformists and members of the congregation at neighbouring Waldringfield. Unfortunately, the chapel does not have any early records, but it is also possible that this is an example of a practice which later became a *cause célèbre* in the Akenham Burial case. Briefly, the vicar of Akenham refused to bury a child on the grounds that it had not been christened. Eventually, a resting place was found in the graveyard of a Dissenters Meeting House in Ipswich. The vicar of Martlesham may have followed the same rule and

John Sheming's death certificate. (Author's collection)

since it is unlikely that Caroline had got round to having her son baptised, the family were faced with a problem of where John should be interred.

Mr Pawson, however, saw no reason why the burial should not take place and gave orders to John Hubbard, his sexton, to dig a grave for a child for burial 'on the first Sabbath in August'. So the funeral was held on 4 August between one and two in the afternoon and was attended by the family and a few friends. It was, as far as Mr Pawson was concerned, a perfectly ordinary funeral. However, a month later, John Hubbard was required to open up the tiny grave and to carry the coffin under the watchful eye of the village police constable to the Red Lion Inn; there to be opened and its contents studied by Mr Moore the surgeon.

It was Mrs Brett who first threw suspicion on to Mary's part in the death of the child. Having played a major role in the last hours of its life, she had, somewhat naturally, discussed the events with her neighbours. Her own husband, who suffered from weak eyesight, then volunteered the information that under two weeks before the death, he had been in John Hudson's general stores in Martlesham when he heard Mary Sheming ask for a pennyworth of arsenic because she was infested with rats. The shopkeeper, who had known Mary for nearly twenty years, warned her as he sold it to be careful where she stored it. Old Mr Brett, who was listening, told her jokingly that she had got enough arsenic in the little packet to put herself to sleep. He then remarked seriously that he hoped she would not poison herself or anybody else. She assured her elderly neighbour that she would sprinkle the poison onto slices of bread and butter and lay them in the shed. She would ensure that it never entered the house at all.

This revelation from her husband added to Mrs Brett's growing suspicions. A fortnight after the burial the gossip had spread throughout the village and come back to Mary, who angrily confronted Mrs Brett, allegedly threatening her that if she did not stop telling lies she would make her very sorry. Mrs Brett tried to calm her down, suggesting that they should sit down and 'have it out', to which Mary had replied, 'Oh no! I'm not saying anything more.' The rumours eventually reached the authorities that little John's death was not necessarily from convulsions, as his death certificate showed, and so an exhumation was ordered, to be followed by an inquest held at Martlesham's Red Lion Inn on 6 September. The surgeon, W.T. Moore, stated that when he examined the body just a month after the death, he found that it was already in an advanced state of decomposition: 'The eyes had disappeared and a blueish and yellowish mould had grown on the face.' Mr Moore, who was assisted by Mr Gissing, then gave details of the results of their examination of the organs of the chest, abdomen and brain. The chest – that is the lungs – was found healthy but the abdomen contained more blood than it should have. The inquest was then adjourned until 14 September for further scientific examination.

Mr Moore, who may not have been called upon before to give evidence in a case involving arsenic poisoning, described in minute detail how he had extracted from the stomach a wine-glassful of a bloody liquid at the bottom of which was almost a teaspoonful of a gritty powder. This he separated from the liquid and placed on a portion of blotting paper. Some of the powder was then heated, producing a smell of garlic. Another portion was placed in a test tube to which was added ammonia nitrate of silver, which produced a reaction of a yellowish precipitation. This particular process was repeated four times with differing amounts, but always with the same result. Ammonia sulphate of copper, deep purplish in colour, was next mixed with the powder and the mixture immediately turned a yellowish green. Mr Moore clearly enjoyed relating his laboratory experiments, for he continued to describe how, when he drew a stick of lunar emetic across another small sample of the powder, it became bright yellow. Next he placed granulated slate into a bent glass tube and then into a phial poured on diluted sulphuric acid, whereby hydrogen gas escaped. When he poured some of the bloody liquid on this, the gas became tainted with an odour of garlic and when he applied a light to the tube, the gas burned with a blue flame. Mr Moore admitted that all the tests he had applied were now considered old fashioned, so he had tried newer methods and he proceeded to expound on these for the benefit of the court. The gist of all this chemical analysis was that the gritty powder found in the baby's stomach was indeed arsenic.

The newspaper reports relating to the findings of the coroner are unusual in that they do not contain any of the written statements of witnesses. It must be assumed that these were sent with other papers to later hearings. What we do have is the summing-up of John Wood, the coroner for the Liberty of St Ethelred, and the signatures of all the members of the jury. Interestingly, one of them, John Buckingham, did not swear the oath on the Bible. Instead he made an affirmation because, we are informed, he was 'of the people called Quakers'. In his report, Mr Wood stated that:

Mary Sheming … not having the fear of God before her eyes but being moved and seduced by the instigation of the Devil and of her malice aforethought contriving and intending with poison feloniously and wilfully to kill the said John … [with] one drachm of arsenic mixed in a certain quantity of mucilaginous liquid to whit a pint … did compel and force the child to take drink and swallow down the poison in the liquid.

Mary appeared at the Woodbridge Quarter Session in October and from there she was remanded in Ipswich Gaol until her trial in December. Throughout this time she maintained her innocence. Unfortunately, instead of gaining public sympathy, she stirred up even more animosity by claiming that one of her daughters was the real culprit. Through the governor of the gaol, she issued a statement that after using three quarters of the arsenic she had purchased for the rats, she had left the remainder in its wrapping in the shed. Later, she had seen fourteen-year-old Elizabeth take it. She had challenged her as to what she had done with it but even after she had flogged her, the girl had still refused to say where she had put it. But the night before the baby died, her daughter Matilda said she had found the packet in a drawer. When the police searched the house, they found only the paper wrapper. Later it was said that the sisters had discussed their mother's possible guilt in the presence of their father and, according to Matilda, when she had asked Elizabeth, 'how do you know it wasn't mother?' Elizabeth had replied she knew it wasn't.

Mary was held in Ipswich Gaol until her trial at the Winter Assizes, which were held on 13 December in the Shire Hall in Bury St Edmunds. Her guilt was almost a foregone conclusion with no new evidence being brought forward by the prosecution and nothing being offered in her defence. When sentence was pronounced, the *Suffolk Chronicle* noted that Mary's eyes held those of her daughter Caroline in a steady gaze. The execution was fixed for Saturday, 11 January 1845.

In some respects, in the four weeks of life left to her, Mary had more opportunity to rest and relax than she probably had ever had. She did not have to consider where the next meal was coming from; indeed she was fed three adequate meals a day. When she felt ill she was able to stay either in the dayroom or in her bed. Her female prison attendants found her both civil and respectful towards them and it appears that over time they came to regard her with sympathy. When the death sentence was pronounced, the judge expressed the desire that during the waiting period before execution the prisoner should have every opportunity to make a full confession of her guilt before God. To this end, it was the duty of the prison chaplain to visit the condemned prisoner daily and to accompany her to her final end. Mary attended chapel with other prisoners just once, but was taken ill during the course of the service and had to be taken back to the day room. It was there or later in her cell that the Revd S.F. Page met her each day to offer what spiritual comfort he could. He worried that he could not get her to admit to her guilt but she was quite willing to join him in prayer. He worried too that there were frequent contradictions and inconsistencies in her narration of the events leading up to the crime of which she was accused; still she persisted in throwing the blame on other members of her family.

Surprisingly, the local magistrates used their powers to allow Mary a number of visitors on different occasions. One of the first was her nineteen-year-old daughter Matilda, who, sometime before Mary, had been brought to trial and herself been sentenced to a term of imprisonment. On Saturday 3 August she had been caught shoplifting in Woodbridge. She had taken a shawl valued at eleven shillings and five yards of ribbon. This was the day before baby John's funeral, so one can't help speculating that she had intended to wear the shawl

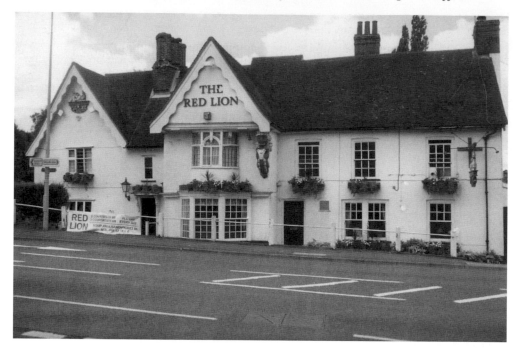

The Red Lion, Martlesham. (Author's collection)

on that occasion. She appeared in court on 16 October and was sentenced to three months imprisonment. For some reason the judge ordered that the first and last weeks of her sentence were to be served in solitary confinement. She was held in a different part of the women's section of the gaol to her mother. She was reputed to have collapsed in a hysterical fit when she had heard of Mary's sentence, and these fits became frequent over the next week or so. Two days before the execution, Matilda was granted a final interview with her mother. It was an excruciatingly painful encounter for both of them. The girl's heart-rending screams as she was led away were heard in every part of the prison. At her going, Mary dropped to her knees and prayed earnestly for her child.

Later that day, Thomas, Caroline and the rest of the children came to make their final goodbyes. Apparently affection was shown on all sides and Caroline, reputedly, told her mother she forgave her. Mary spent the following day talking with the chaplain and her attendants. In spite of remonstrations from the Revd Page she still maintained her innocence and when told that she could not take the sacrament of Holy Communion until she was in a state of penance, she accepted that it must be so and the chaplain did not press the point further. Mary then slept from midnight until five on Saturday morning. As she slept, the prison officials were busy preparing the scaffold.

Saturday 11 January dawned darkly with a steady downpour of rain. Outside the gaol, in spite of the dismal weather, a crowd began to gather. By noon it was estimated that between 5,000 and 6,000 people had crammed themselves into St Helen's Street for the spectacle. The local constabulary was on standby for any trouble that might occur. Inside the gaol, Mary was preparing herself by praying with the chaplain, Mrs Johnson (the wife of the gaoler who acted as matron of the women's quarters) and the attendants who had been with her throughout

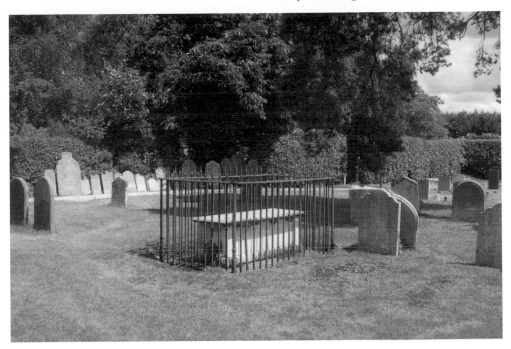

The graveyard of Waldringfield Baptist Church. (Author's collection)

her stay. However calm Mary appeared to be, her equanimity was shaken when the screaming of Matilda reached her and she fainted. As she recovered her senses, she was heard to say, 'my wicked children have brought their mother's grey hairs with sorrow to the grave.'

By 11.50 a.m. the hangman, William Calcraft, had arrived from Newgate ready to perform the execution. Mary, wearing a blue and white day gown and a white cap with a deep border, was led out from the women's day room and down the principal staircase to the ground floor, where she met Calcraft. She showed surprise when he put his hand on her arm to help her. Taking her leave of Mrs Johnson and the nurse who had cared for her, she shed no tears, but both the other two women were greatly overcome with emotion. Mrs Johnson in fact withdrew to her private apartments. Now that the hanging was imminent this was indeed a highly charged moment – the reality of what was to happen affected all the staff. None of them had seen a woman executed during their working lives, for Mary was the first woman to hang in Ipswich Gaol since Elizabeth Woolterton thirty years before (*see* Chapter One).

The little procession halted in the turnkey's room so that Mary's arms could be pinioned. She was seated on a stool while her hands and arms were bound. Suddenly she looked about her wildly, exclaiming, 'oh dear, oh dear.' The next moment she had regained her mental composure, concentrating instead on the pressure of the cords upon her wrists. No doubt her arms had become very thin in the last few weeks for Calcraft carefully loosened the bonds slightly. Next he pulled the wide border on her cap right down over her eyes and to her chin. Mary had previously requested that she be blindfolded before she ascended the scaffold so that she would not have to see the crowd. But now she complained that she couldn't breathe and said she had expected her eyes to be covered with a handkerchief. She asked for Mrs Johnson, hoping that lady would understand and come to her aid, but she was no longer there.

The chaplain led the way up the steps to the platform, reading the most beautiful parts of the burial service, but as Mary followed him, the hem of her dress got caught and Calcraft had to halt to release it. Then he positioned her under the beam and adjusted the rope. Mary called out to him, 'Pull up my cap, I want to see the people.' Calcraft chose to ignore her request and left the platform knife in hand, ready to cut the rope that secured it. Mary remained with her bound hands as if in prayer. The chaplain had continued with his prayers, still hoping that at the very last minute she would confess her great sin. But her only words were, 'Oh God, be merciful to me a sinner for Christ's sake, Amen.' The chaplain dropped a handkerchief and left the platform and Calcraft cut the rope.

Concerned readers of the *Ipswich Journal* would have been pleased to learn that such was Mr Calcraft's expertise that Mary appeared to suffer little, for her neck was dislocated instantly by the fall and life was extinct in two minutes. The body was left hanging for an hour to send a moral message to the crowd. It was also reported that the crowd had behaved reasonably well but that there had been little sympathy for the woman. Calcraft's last task was to remove the body ready for burial within the gaol, then, with his fee of twelve guineas, he boarded the evening coach for London.

Was Mary Sheming guilty? If so, then she was even more despicable in trying to place the blame on to one of her children. If she wasn't, then the question remains, who did put the arsenic in the baby's food?

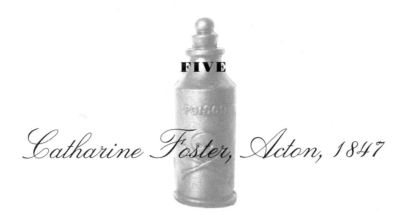

FIVE

Catharine Foster, Acton, 1847

One of the problems one comes across when dealing with trial cases from over 200 years ago is that no one is reported at the time as having asked the right questions. Hearsay evidence may have been given in passing but no one in court directly asked Catharine Foster why, after only three weeks of marriage, she felt compelled to murder her new husband, particularly as she was absent from him for almost two weeks out of that three. Of all the murders committed in Suffolk's history, Catharine's crime ranks alongside the brutal murder of Maria Marten in the Red Barn at Polstead as being one of the most written about. I make no apology for including a retelling here, for it is just possible that a female viewpoint may throw a different light on the case.

Quite apart from any human interest Catharine's story may have, it was in some respects a turning point in the history of criminal justice. For the trial for murder of the barely seventeen year old country girl aroused great public interest nationally. By the 1840s there was a growing repugnance at the idea of capital punishment, which was fuelled in this case not only by the prospect of so young a woman being hanged but also that executions were made an occasion for public spectacle.

Catharine Morley, as she was known prior to her married life, lived in the village of Acton in west Suffolk, three miles north east of the small market town of Sudbury and about fourteen miles from the bustling town of Bury St Edmunds. In the 1840s Acton was described as a pleasant village with a population of 550, with most of the men and boys employed on the land. There was one inn, the Crown, and an attractive church, All Saints', the incumbent at that time being the Revd Lawrence Ottley. Unusually for the period, Acton already had a National School, built under the auspices of 'The National Society for the Education of the Poor according to the principles of the Church of England', which had been opened in 1839. Catharine therefore had at least four years' education and although she might not have been the brightest of pupils, she had certainly learned to read and write, though spelling, as we shall see later, was not her strongest subject. She would have spoken with the rounded accent of Suffolk that made her write her Christian name on her marriage certificate as she pronounced it, 'Catharine'.

When the census was taken in 1841, the Morley household consisted of Catharine's father Robert, aged sixty-two, who was listed as a pensioner, which means he had at one time been either a soldier or sailor. In civilian life he had made a living as a 'hawker' trading goods from door-to-door. His first wife, Ellen, had produced five children in the ten years before her death,

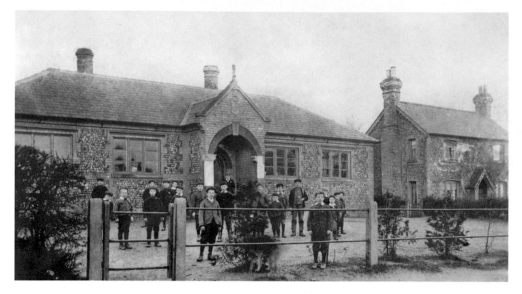

Acton School. (Reproduced by kind permission of Roger Lane)

the youngest of whom was still under a year old when Robert married Maria Brewster, who was twenty-seven years his junior. Together they had a further seven children, although by 1841 only daughters Catharine (eleven), Sarah (nine), Hannah (six) and three-year-old son Thomas were living with their parents in Acton Lane, in the middle cottage of a row of three which had been carved out of one original dwelling. Their neighbours, Mr and Mrs Simpson, occupied the left-hand cottage and to the right of them was William Pawsey, a farm labourer who lived with his granddaughter, Mary Ann Chinery. As was usual at that time, the gardens of each property were ill-defined; where animals – and children – roamed freely. The midden, or dung heap, was situated in the ditch below a hedge, which formed the boundary with farmland.

In the year following the census, Robert Morley died and it became necessary for Maria to find ways to support the family. She was probably already employed locally as a washerwoman but as time passed she increased her workload, attending the larger households of farmers and gentry over a fairly wide area, where she would spend entire days doing the laundry. This meant she left home very early in the morning and returned quite late in the day, depending on the time of year. Apart from the wage she earned, it was part of her contract that she would be fed. This was a decided bonus as it meant she had one less mouth to feed at home and as soon as they were old enough, the two older girls went into living-in service, thus lessening her burden.

Catharine was still a schoolgirl of twelve or thirteen when she first caught the eye of John Foster, who was seven years her senior. One might speculate on what sort of young man approaching his twenties spent time hanging around waiting for the opportunity to talk to her. However, Catharine's attraction was such that even before she left school at fourteen, John had, so we are led to believe, told her mother that he would like to marry her. Mrs Morley had sensibly told him that the girl was far too young to think of marriage, but John had indicated he was willing to wait.

On leaving school, Catharine became a living-in maid to a Mr Wade of Great Waldingfield. This village was about two and a half miles from John's home, but on Sundays he attended the church there so that he could walk Catharine back to her employer's home after the service. He continued to court her when she took up new employment in Bulmer, where her sister was also in service. For John this now meant a walk of between nine and ten miles from his home and back. However, afterwards he would take the opportunity to call in on Mrs Morley to tell her how both her daughters were. During the week, Catharine, who obviously enjoyed writing, wrote him letters that led him to believe that she returned his affection. They were found after his death amongst his belongings. John was unable to write his name but perhaps he could read enough to understand her letters.

At the end of September 1846, Catharine was dismissed from her post and had to return home, a situation that did not please her mother. However, the situation meant that at last the girl would have the opportunity to accept a long-standing invitation to go and stay for a few days with her aunt in Pakenham, a few miles away on the other side of Bury St Edmunds, so arrangements for this were put in hand.

But John had another plan. It appears that during his Sunday evening visits to Mrs Morley, he had suggested he might move into her house as a lodger. Mrs Morley had questioned the propriety of this, but with Catharine's unemployment John now saw this as his opportunity to hasten the marriage and so, with her mother's consent, as she was under age, the service took place at All Saints' Church, Acton, on Wednesday 28 October. Weddings then were very simple affairs, even the church ceremony itself was witnessed by very few. The bridegroom's mother and sisters, for example, did not attend the service, though they did join the bridal pair at the bride's home for a simple wedding breakfast. Following the wedding, the newlyweds settled themselves into Mrs Morley's house, an arrangement that suited her well as it meant a steady weekly wage coming into the house with her son-in-law. John was also anxious to leave his

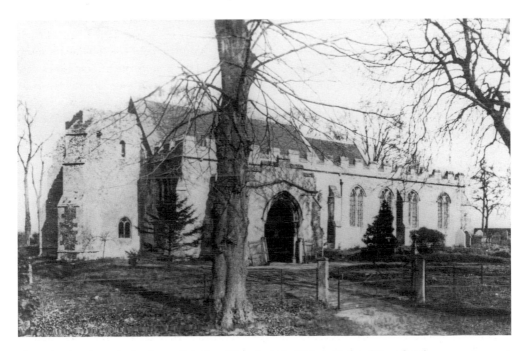

Acton church as it was in the nineteenth century. (Reproduced by kind permission of Roger Lane)

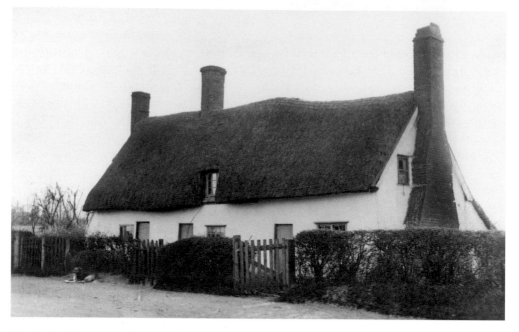

The Morleys' Home – middle section of the cottage. (Reproduced by kind permission of Roger Lane)

own home as it was somewhat noisy and overcrowded, for two of his unmarried sisters had small children, delightfully described by his new mother-in-law as 'chance children'.

Having successfully won his bride and made her legally his property on the Wednesday, is difficult to understand why he was willing 'to give his permission' for her to go and visit her aunt just three days later? When he saw her off in the Carrier's cart for Bury St Edmunds on the Saturday morning, he was heard to tell her she could stay a month. There is no way to tell how this remark was made, if it ever was. It could have been in the soft tones of a lover willing to indulge his new wife's every whim, or it could have been shouted in anger – as far as he was concerned she could be away as long as she liked. However, Catharine was reputed to have replied that she would be back in two weeks. One can imagine several different reasons why he may have been amenable to her going. Perhaps the most obvious is that having got what he wanted, a wife and a new home, John was more interested in his personal comfort than the joys of marital bliss, which may not have lived up to expectation anyway. Certainly, had Catharine been so deeply attached to him, she would not have left so soon, even for the great pleasure of seeing the bright lights of Bury St Edmunds and beyond. A perhaps more unlikely, though feasible, suggestion is that by the time he came to be married, John had lost interest in Catharine but quite fancied her mother, with whom he seems to have been on very good terms. Mrs Morley was still physically attractive and indeed she found herself another husband the following year. It is also possible that Catharine was pregnant and, not wishing to start married life with an encumbrance – and we already know John's attitude to babies in the house – she intended to use her visit to deal with the situation. That might well account for her purchase of a small quantity of arsenic, which was thought by some to be an abortifacient. Whatever the real reason, it has to be agreed that it was a decidedly odd situation.

Unfortunately, no information has come to light about Catharine's stay in Pakenham. We do not know either her aunt's name or why neither the prosecution nor the defence believed that she could contribute anything to the case. Nowadays she would be regarded as vital in being able to throw light on Catharine's behaviour during the time they were together. If aunt and niece were close, then presumably they would have talked and Catharine might have confided any misgivings she had about her new husband. It has been suggested that Catharine really loved another young man who had left the area and for whom she had gone in search. No evidence was ever produced that there was such a young man and without doubt someone would have been able to name him. A witness later testified that Catharine had told her that while she was away she had discovered just how easy it was to find employment in Bury St Edmunds and that had she known that, she would not have married. This is the sort of chance remark one young woman might make to another but it is hardly proof that she intended to kill her husband.

During the time that she was away, John, who showed no signs of pining for his new wife, continued with his work at a farm in nearby Chilton. The only event of any significance took place in the early part of the first week when he and his fellow labourers, James Pleasance and William Steed, were engaged in loading trusses of hay from a stack onto a horse-drawn wagon. John's position was on top of the wagon and when one of the trusses slipped and fell, it brought him down with it. Steed was concerned that he was hurt but John had assured him he was all right.

The two weeks passed and Catharine came home on the Saturday as she had promised and her younger sister, Hannah, went to Pakenham in her place. No one could remember later what sort of reunion had taken place between husband and wife, indeed the only memorable thing was that John's sister, Susan, said he had told her he had a headache when they walked home from church on Sunday. (Much was made later of what a religious young man he was.) John went off to work on the Monday and Tuesday, taking, as was customary, some bread to eat when the labourers stopped for their breakfast at half past ten and dinner at about three thirty. His friend Steed testified that, apart from mentioning his headache, John had seemed in very good spirits at the time and was a strong and healthy young man.

Catharine and John's marriage certificate. (Reproduced by kind permission of Sudbury Register Office & OPSI)

On the Tuesday Catharine walked the mile and a half from her home to visit her mother-in-law. She stayed long enough to join the family there for dinner but left about four o'clock when, bearing in mind the time of year, the daylight began fading. She mentioned to Mrs Foster that she was leaving then in order to get a pudding on to boil. Mrs Foster, who had been in the habit of giving her son a boiled suet pudding or dumpling every night for his supper when he came home from work, enquired if Catharine was doing the same. Her new daughter-in-law replied that she had not done so far.

For the sequence of events that followed Catharine's arrival home that evening we have to rely on the testimony of her brother, Thomas, a child of nine. He had spent the day at school where, as he later told the judge, he was learning to read from the Bible and to spell from Carpenter's spelling book. School started at nine and finished at five. During the midday break he had come home to get himself some bread and butter that Catharine had left out for him. When he came in after school he found his sister was at home and he watched her as she prepared dumplings, noting that she used her own flour in the kneading trough and not his mother's. It was Thomas's testimony at the inquest which threw suspicion upon Catharine, for he said that after she had mixed the two dumplings, she had taken a screw of paper from her pocket and emptied a dark powder into the mixing bowl. She had then thrown the paper into the fire. This would account for why, when the house was searched later, no trace of arsenic was found. Thomas was not a reliable witness, later changing his story to omit the reference to the dark powder. According to Thomas, he and Catharine shared the dumpling that was cooked straight in the boiler, while the second, larger one, was wrapped in a cloth and left for John. The boy had sat beside the fire with his plate on his lap to eat his part of the dumpling with some potatoes. In Thomas's version of events Catharine had just served out her own meal when John came in.

John had left work at six o'clock and walked home with James Pleasance. He seemed in very good spirits and sang as they walked along, thus confirming the general belief that there was nothing wrong in the marriage. John came in and greeted Catharine before going into the yard to wash his hands and face before eating. He then sat down at the table beside his wife and started tucking into the second dumpling, almost finishing it. But it was not long before he complained of heartburn and then had to rush out into the backyard, where he was violently sick.

Catharine had seemed solicitous in following her husband outside as he vomited. She probably even helped him into a bed in a small ground floor room, which was where Mrs Morley found him on her return from her day's work some time after seven o'clock. She immediately took charge of the situation and turned her hand to emptying the basins of dark-stained vomit into the ditch adjoining the garden. By this time John was suffering from both severe sickness and diarrhoea and was very weak. So concerned for him was Mrs Morley that she sent Catharine to buy six-pennyworth of brandy. This she mixed into freshly made oatmeal gruel, which she hoped would settle John's stomach. Unfortunately, it did not have the effect she hoped for, for that too was quickly brought back. Mrs Morley then asked John's permission for Catharine to share her bed that night so that he could get some rest. Both women got up throughout the night to attend to him but by morning Mrs Morley felt they ought to have medical help. At around eight o'clock Catharine set off to walk to Mr Jones's surgery in Long Melford, a journey of two miles yet, according to Mr Jones, it was nearly 10 a.m. by the time she arrived. When she described John as suffering from a bowel complaint, he assumed it was a case of the English Cholera and prescribed the usual medication of mercury with chalk and rhubarb in the form of two powders. Catharine told him that John wished him to call and the doctor said he would. Catharine forgot to mention to Mr Jones that John was now her husband, though she did remember to tell him he was living in her mother's cottage.

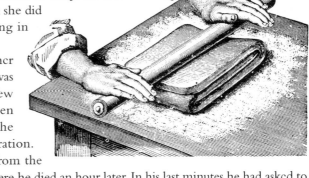

By the time she reached home, her mother had left for work and John was very ill indeed. During the next few hours he grew much worse. When Mrs Morley came back at three she was horrified by his rapid deterioration. In making an attempt to get up from the bed John collapsed in her arms, where he died an hour later. In his last minutes he had asked to see his mother and sisters, but there was no one to send for them. It was also said later that even in his very weak state he had asked Catharine to join him in prayer. As only Catharine and Mrs Morley were present throughout, one wonders where that piece of information came from. Mr Jones arrived some time later and, though surprised at the speed of death, had no suspicion that anything other than the English Cholera was responsible for it.

It is one of the ironies of crime stories – both in fact and fiction – that it is often some insignificant detail which is the undoing of the perpetrator. In this case it was chickens wandering from the farmer's land into the boundary ditch. There, foraging among the fallen leaves, they found the remnants of John Morley's undigested meal and the scrap of dumpling that had been thrown out, which Mrs Simpson from next door had found and carefully crumbled up for them. The day after John died, a number of chickens were found dead. When their crops were examined and found to contain both traces of dumpling and arsenic, suspicions were aroused, although when Mr Jones performed his post-mortem on John, he still thought his original diagnosis was correct, though he did also discover that one of the deceased's main arteries had ruptured. Just to be on the safe side, he had removed the stomach and part of the intestines for safekeeping. When the coroner's inquest took place on Saturday at the Crown Inn, the doctor was ordered to send the specimens for analysis to the best authority on the subject, Mr Image of Bury St Edmunds. In the meantime John was buried in Acton churchyard but within days, the grave was re-opened, the coffin removed and a full examination carried out on the corpse. When more than minor traces of arsenic were found in the body, the police moved in to search the cottage. The pudding cloth and flour that Catharine had used were taken away for tests. These, plus the other forensic revelations and the evidence given at the inquest, were sufficient for Catharine to be charged with the murder of her husband.

She was held in Bury Gaol until her trial at the assizes at the end of March. On the last day of the trial, a Saturday, the judge spent two hours summing up but the jury took just a quarter of an hour to reach their verdict of 'guilty'. According to the press reports, 'the prisoner, on hearing the verdict, betrayed no symptoms of emotion.' When she was brought back into court for sentencing on the Monday, the judge told her:

It is my melancholy duty to pronounce the sentence of the law against you that requires that your life be forfeited for the crime you have committed. I would advise you to make the utmost use of the short time you will remain in this world. Seek peace and mercy where

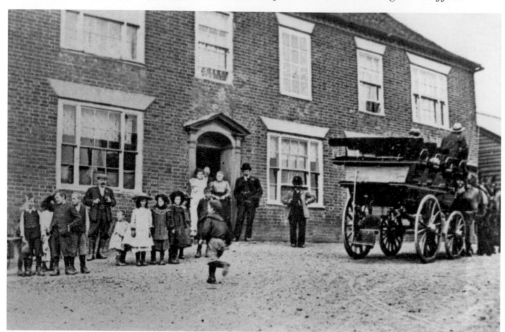

The Crown Inn, Acton. (Reproduced by kind permission of Roger Lane)

now alone you will be able to find them … it remains to me but to pass the judgement of the law, that you may be taken from this place from which you came and hence to the place of execution and there to be hanged by the neck until you are dead and that your body be buried in the precincts of the prison in which you shall be confined. And may the Lord in his infinite mercy have compassion on your soul.

Even as she listened to the words of the judge she seemed almost unmoved, merely applying a handkerchief to her eyes at the conclusion. However, the paper did report that they understood that she had later been more affected but not in a very great degree.

The execution was ordered for Saturday 17 April 1847. During the two weeks left before that date, petitions or 'memorials' were circulated on her behalf. One was for the recognition that the general principle of capital punishment was un-Christian, the second was a plea for mercy in her particular case, and the third was a petition for mercy to the Queen from the women of Bury and its vicinity. None bore fruit.

The power of the press was just as strong in the past as it is today and the *Bury and Norwich Post* lent its wholehearted support to the cause for the abolition of capital punishment. The day before the execution, it reported that there had been no response to the petitions and in its comment column it stated:

It is all but certain that before this meets the eye of our readers the unfortunate girl will have paid the extreme penalty of the law. A few more questions and more agitation of the public mind upon this question [Capital Punishment] and the blot upon our civilisation will be removed. On Friday, we are informed that disquieting piece of religious mockery, the condemned sermon, is to be delivered, the privilege of witnessing the farce is to be confined to prison officers. The order is preaching on Friday afternoon and strangling on Saturday morning and we fear we must add, drinking on Saturday evening. Surely wise statesmen must ere long change the law which is so brutalizing in its effects. We freely confess we have less patience with their tardiness than with the obstinacy of the fanatic who thinks the disgusting exhibition is of Divine appointment. However grovelling his notions may be of the Deity, he acts upon his own ideas of right and his mental darkness …

As with today's newspaper reports, we have to wonder from what source such detailed information was garnered. The account of Catharine's last hours was slanted to make the most of the paper's stance on capital punishment. It started with the arresting statement, 'the wretched woman was strangled according to law in front of Bury Gaol. The previous day the sermon by the Revd C.J.P. Eyre was from Numbers xxxii, 23 – Ye have sinned against the Lord. Be sure your sins will find you out.'

The rector of Acton, the Revd J. Ottley, who visited Catharine regularly during her period of imprisonment, made his final visit on Friday, during which time he suggested that the Bible he had given her on her wedding day should be sent on her behalf to her mother-in-law as a memento of John. When he left, the chaplain, the Revd Eyre, remained with her until ten in the evening. She then retired to bed but slept only fitfully until half past one in the morning. After that sleep seemed impossible so she passed the dark hours in devotional reading. Mr Eyre arrived very early to remain by her side until the end. When the summons came for her to leave her room, she broke down in tears but with the reverend's comfort and support she

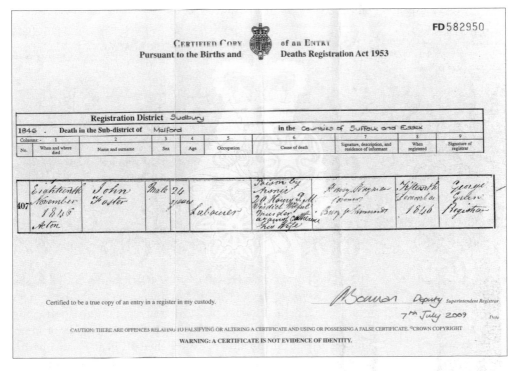

John Foster's death certificate. (*Reproduced by kind permission of Sudbury Register office & OPSI*)

managed to regain her composure, and it was noted that after she had been through the process of pinioning, she walked with an extraordinary firmness across the yards to the turnkey's lodge and up the stairs to its flat roof and so to the iron door, outside which stood the scaffold.

She appeared before the vast crowd, estimated at around 10,000, at precisely nine o'clock. She was said to have looked out at the heaving mass of humanity with surprising calm. But when the governor of the gaol, to whom she had earlier expressed the desire to address the crowd, asked her if she wanted to say anything, she replied, 'No, I thank you sir, I can't speak.' Calcraft, the executioner, adjusted the rope and at the signal, the drop fell. Her limbs contorted for a minute or two, during which time two men who were at the foot of the gallows began shouting, 'Shame! Murder!' The *Bury Post* reporter was appalled by this display. It transpired that the two men in question were 'two persons who had come down on behalf of the *London Weekly Press* and who had applied, in a state very unfitted for the purpose, to be admitted into the prison.' Excessive drinking among journalists was obviously frowned upon in Bury St Edmunds and our anonymous Suffolk chronicler felt that the reputation of the press had been impugned. He was also quick to refute the suggestion later made by the Marquis of Westmeath, who discussed the case in the House of Lords, that Calcraft had been negligent and caused Catharine unnecessary suffering. It seems that Catharine was not as light in weight as her figure suggested.

The reporter now played his trump card. He was able to reproduce for the first time a letter and extracts from a confession written by Catharine in her last days. When a prisoner, having pleaded innocence, was found guilty by the jury, it was the duty of the prison governor to persuade the prisoner to make a full written confession of guilt in order to ease their conscience before death. In the case of those who were illiterate the governor would take down the confession for them. Catharine wrote her first confession herself and it was reproduced in the paper exactly as she had written it, the reporter commenting only that it showed an example of her education:

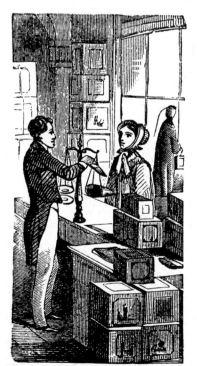

Now sir first of all I must confess that I ame gilty veary gilty of this awful criame and well dearserves the death that I ame condemned to die and as I ame soane to steand before my hevvenly Judg I wish to Speake the truth, and I ame veary sorey to say I bought it and did it my own sealf and I did deni it till this veary day and I did not wish to get clear for if I had I neaver should have been hapy and now I trust I shall be hapy in heven sir do not Show it to any wone wile I ame on this side of the grave but after I ame gone I wish all to know it is riten veary bad sir but I did as I could.

Catharine Foster

However, this was not the only confession she made and on 12 April she gave more concrete details. Now she wrote that she had bought the poison from the chemist's shop in Sudbury. Since she had often been into the shop on errands for her mistress, Mr Eley, the proprietor, knew her, but on this occasion she had been served by his young male assistant. She had, she said, visited the shop three days before she mixed it in the dumplings. This

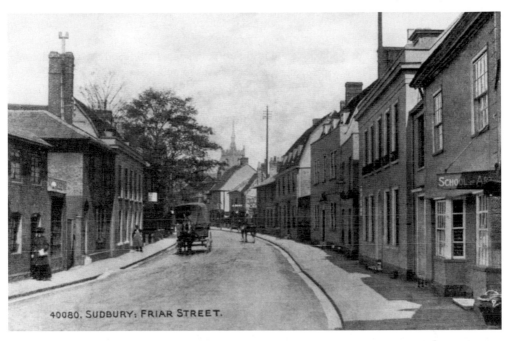

40080. SUDBURY: FRIAR STREET.

Above and below: *Sudbury street scenes. (Reproduced by kind permission of Roger Lane)*

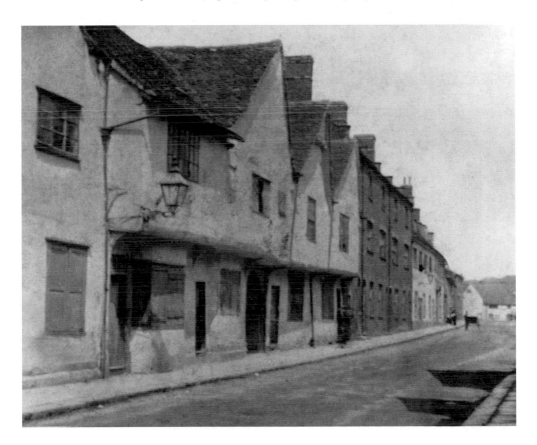

would have been on the Saturday, the day she returned from Pakenham. If she had already made up her mind while she was away to kill John, then why did she not make the purchase in Bury? It seems strange that she would have come home and then immediately walked to Sudbury to buy it unless something had occurred when she reached home that made her take the sudden decision. On the other hand, if she had wanted arsenic for an abortion, it was likely that she had bought it much earlier and still had some in her possession. The trial never sought to establish how she had come by the arsenic.

On another day she confessed that no one had persuaded her to kill John and no one knew of her intention to do so. She also said her husband had always been good and kind but that she had no affection for him and wished that she could go back into service.

Then there was the mystery of the letter. When Catharine's body was prepared for burial, a letter was discovered tucked in the bosom of her dress. It was said that she had believed she would go to the grave in what she was wearing, so it was thought that she intended this letter to go with her. Which raises the question why did she write it if it were not intended to be read? It was addressed to her mother. This time the spelling had been corrected for publication:

My Dear Mother, I never wrote a letter to you with so much joy and pleasure in all the letters I have wrote to you as this. Dear Mother you know that I never had any wish to live and I wish it had pleased the Lord to call me before I had known anything but My Dear Mother while the lamp holds out to burn the worst sinner may return. I hope you will make yourself happy about me, for I am going to a better place than being in this world of trouble and I wish I had been there ten years ago, but I am glad to come to it at last. My Dear Mother I had every attendance that ever could be for both body and soul. That dear Mrs James [the turnkey's wife] have behaved to me like a mother. If my life could have been spared I did not wish for it. That is from the bottom of my heart. I have a great hope that I am going to Heaven and there

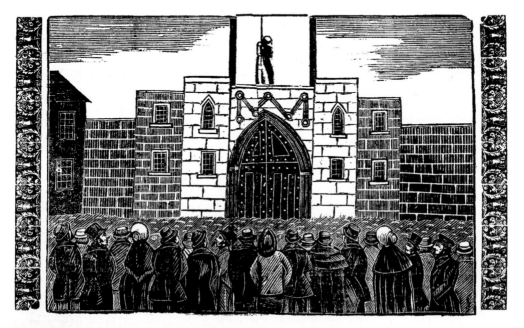

The hanging of Catharine Foster. (Reproduced by kind permission of SRO/Bury)

to see my Saviour face to face, and also that other dear creature I have injured: and the years I might have spent in pleasure with him on earth, I hope I shall rest with him in Heaven.

The letter was unsigned but was dated 17 April. The source of this 'leaked' letter said her attendants had declared that she did not write it during the night or in the early morning. It was true, they said, that she had several times started writing but she had then burned the papers. Somehow it seems she had managed to secrete this piece. Perhaps she intended to give it to the chaplain to hand on to her mother, to whom she had said farewell days before. The religious tone of the letter shows the strong influence of the clerical gentlemen who had spent time with her. It is a pity we do not know the significance, if any, of the reference to her possible death ten years earlier. But there is something about the second half of the final sentence that just does not ring true.

Once the execution was over, the huge crowds dispersed to the numerous inns and alehouses to discuss over pints of ale what they had seen. Drinking continued throughout the day and there was, it was said, as much merriment in the streets as if it were a fair day. Most of those who enjoyed 'the holiday' were from out of town, simple folk for whom the spectacle added a bit of colour to an otherwise drab life. A public execution had always been considered a way of teaching the public a moral lesson and for that reason children were brought by their parents to witness the awful fate that awaited wrongdoers. It was to take another hundred years before capital punishment was abolished, but the awful sight of Catharine hanging did achieve one result: she was the last woman to be publicly hanged in Bury.

How odd that a simple seventeen-year-old Suffolk girl should have earned a place in history, even though we still do not know why she put the arsenic in the dumplings. One of the last remarks about her that appeared in the *Bury Post* stated: 'Catharine Foster was always considered a girl of moron and obstinate disposition and phlegmatic temperament but was apt in learning at school and gave satisfaction during the greater part of the time she was in service.' The word 'moron' was at that time an accepted medical classification for someone with a mental age in the range of seven to twelve years, whose communication and social skills prevented them from achieving a certain level of education or undertake employment. Could it be that Catharine enjoyed being in service, where she was told what to do, and that she also enjoyed the 'walking-out' with John but when faced with the reality of a marital relationship she just could not cope?

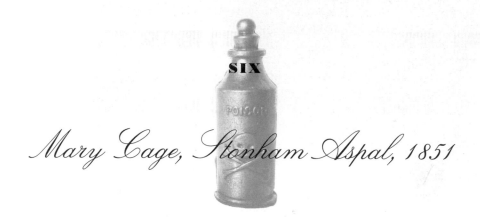

SIX

Mary Cage, Stonham Aspal, 1851

For over 500 years the crime of petty treason was enforced. This was applied to a man who killed his master and to a woman who murdered her husband. A guilty servant was hanged but for the guilty wife the punishment was burning at the stake. Petty treason disappeared from the statute book in 1828, at which time guilty wives were hanged instead. The use of the word 'treason' defines the legal role of a wife in relation to her husband – she was his subject. This may help to explain why the women in this book seemed to be treated more harshly than the men.

Mary and James Cage fit the stereotypical picture of the nineteenth-century agricultural class. Both were born in the village of Stonham Aspal, from which they were rarely absent and where, fifty-six years later, James was to meet his death. James's family was employed on the land and he automatically followed suit. Mary's shoemaker father on the other hand was a skilled tradesman. Neither John nor Mary, who was born in March 1805, received any form of education, so when they married a couple of months after Mary's seventeenth birthday in 1822, both had to make their mark in the marriage register in place of a signature. Their first child, Mary Ann, arrived a few short months later.

As the family grew so it became more difficult to make ends meet. Life was hard and not made any easier for Mary by James's volatile temper. Neighbours testified to the stormy nature of the Cages' marriage, so it came as no surprise that Mary sought affection elsewhere and may explain why their son James, born a couple of years after Mary Ann, was later referred to as Cage's stepson. Over the years life with Cage became so intolerable that twice during the three years preceding his death she left him. In April 1850, Mary ran away with a local man named Robert Tricker and they set up home in a village just outside Ipswich. Two months later, when Mary was shopping in the town, she had the misfortune to encounter her husband in the street. The ensuing fracas that took place led to James being charged with assaulting his wife and being sentenced to a prison term of two months. Mary's freedom was also over as she then had to return home to look after the family, which at that time included Sybilla, her unmarried daughter of nineteen, who was pregnant.

On 7 March 1851 James, his twenty-one-year-old son Richard, and a fellow labourer were working in the fields of a local farm. During the course of the day, James, who was in his mid-fifties, was taken ill with bouts of vomiting and purging. Despite feeling very unwell he had continued to work out the day. He struggled on but three days later, there being no

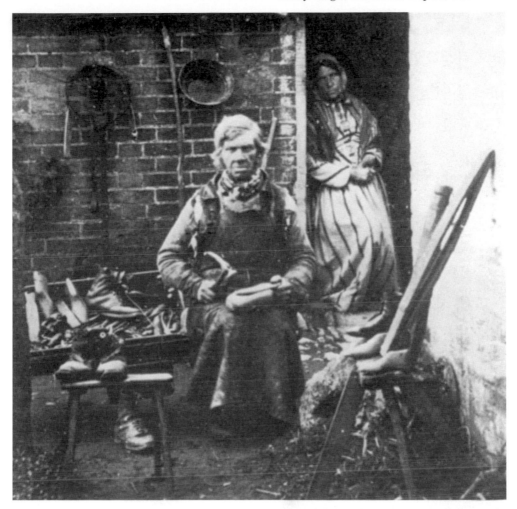

Mary Cage's father was a shoemaker. (Robert Burrows. Reproduced by kind permission of SRO/Ipswich)

improvement in his health, he took to his bed with a very high temperature, complaining of rheumatic pains and a general feeling of lassitude. The following day, Mary called at the surgery of Mr E.R. Lock of Debenham to ask him to call and see her husband. She explained that James was suffering from a bowel complaint so Mr Lock gave her the standard remedy used in such cases, but whether this was in powder, pill or liquid form the surgeon was later unable to remember. When he visited on the 12th he diagnosed James's condition to be of a rheumatic nature, for which he prescribed a fever mixture. Mary walked to the surgery – a distance of four miles – on both the following days to collect further doses of the fever mixture.

Then, on 17 March, Mary made a surprise call on her childhood friend Elizabeth Lambert. When she had parted from her own husband some five years earlier, Elizabeth had lodged with the Cages for four months, so she was well aware of the stormy nature of their marriage. Elizabeth earned her living as a washerwoman and nurse and for the past year she had lived in Debenham, acting as a full time carer to the bedridden Mrs Parker. Although Mary had to

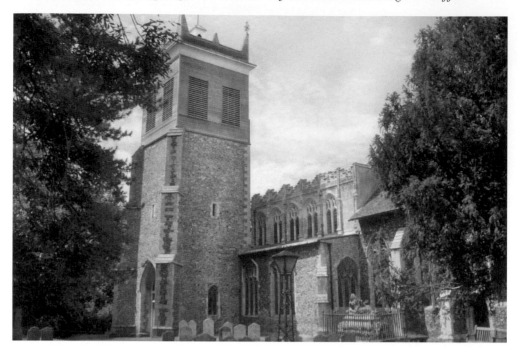

The Church of St Mary and St Lambert, Stonham Aspal. (Author's collection)

come to Debenham on several occasions recently, this was the first time she had called. When, after an hour or so of exchanging news and gossip, it was time for Mary to leave, Elizabeth walked some of the way towards the village with her. As they went along, Mary confided that her married daughter, Mary Ann, was plagued with rats and mice in her cottage and wondered if Elizabeth would mind going to the shop for her to buy a pennyworth of the stuff to deal with them. Later, Elizabeth testified that she had been reluctant to do so but had eventually agreed and, taking the penny Mary had thrust upon her, she duly asked Mr Smith, the shopkeeper, for 'the stuff'. He had at first refused to supply her but finally he gave her a packet of what Elizabeth thought looked like an ash-coloured powder. Mindful of his legal duty, Mr Smith cautioned Elizabeth about its use and wrote something on the packet. When she handed it to Mary, Elizabeth, being unable to read, asked what the words said and was told it said 'rank poison'.

Walking the four miles home, Mary willingly accepted a lift in a passing cart driven by William Gunn, a painter and glazier, who chatted with her throughout the journey. Noticing she had a medicine bottle in her basket, he asked who was ill. When she told him it was her husband, he asked her jokingly how she would manage if he died, to which she had replied, 't'other man is not far off.' Gunn took this to be a light-hearted reply and certainly did not get the impression that his passenger had either any weighty problem on her mind nor did she appear to be in any hurry to get home.

Two days later, Mr Lock again visited and found James still in bed and no better. On that occasion, as on the second out of the three visits he made to the house, Lock found Mary to be absent, so he left word for her to collect medicine from the surgery the next day, which she did. The following day one of James's sons took him a slice of bread and butter. Instead of eating

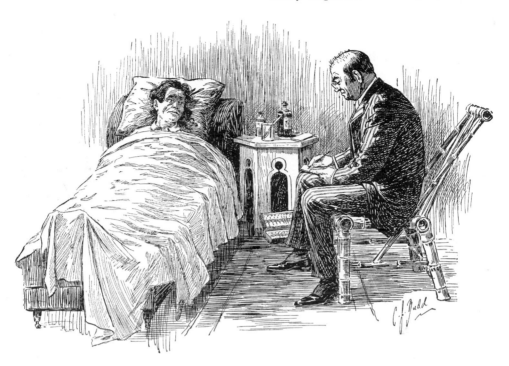

it the man took it and laid it against his stomach, as if in an effort to get some relief from the acute physical irritation he was experiencing in his abdomen. The pain had become so intense that his nails had gouged strips of flesh from his stomach. Equally strong was the itching in his gums, which in a frenzied attempt to alleviate he scratched so deeply that not only did the gums bleed but he had also torn flesh from his mouth. When Samuel Oxborrow, a shoemaker and long time neighbour of the Cages, called to see how James was, he was horrified to witness this. In between the bouts of scratching, James told Samuel that he felt so bad in his stomach and mouth that he just didn't know what to do. His behaviour frightened the visitor, who thought the sick man was going mad, especially when he started searching his bed supposedly for ferrets.

Oxborrow told his wife Kezia what he had seen and she decided she would use the excuse to visit Sybilla and her new baby and see for herself the situation in the Cages' household. She found Mary sitting disconsolately by a meagre fire. When Kezia asked after James, Mary had replied that he was no better. She was perhaps by this time so worn out with nursing him that her remarks that he was a very wicked man and that she prayed to God to take him before morning may be taken as those of a woman at the end of her patience. It was only later that Kezia was to read more into those words – and the fact that Mary had ignored James when he called to her from upstairs. However, when James had fallen out of bed, Mary had stirred herself to go up and help him back.

When Mr Lock visited around 1 p.m. on Friday 21 March, he found James trying to get out of bed and so delusional that he was unable to give him any rational answers. The doctor told Mary to send for medication during the afternoon, but no one came for it. Samuel Oxborrow called again on the Saturday and was horrified to find that James had deteriorated so much overnight that he no longer recognised him. Like most of his neighbours, Samuel knew poverty,

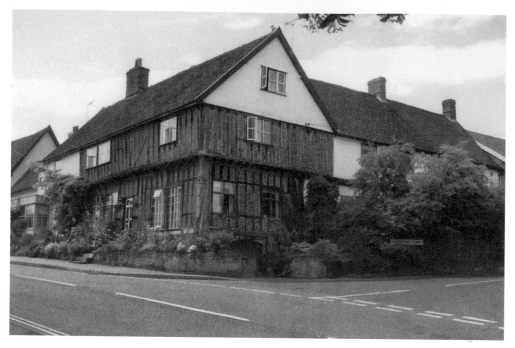

Debenham High Street. (Author's collection)

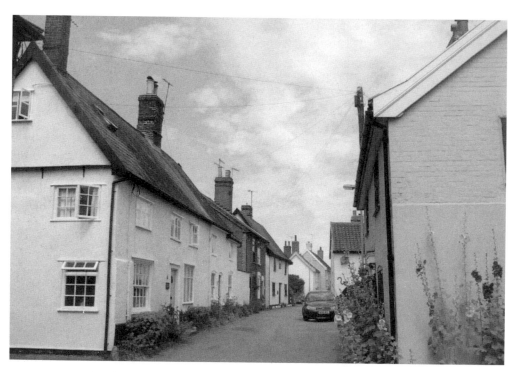

Debenham. (Author's collection)

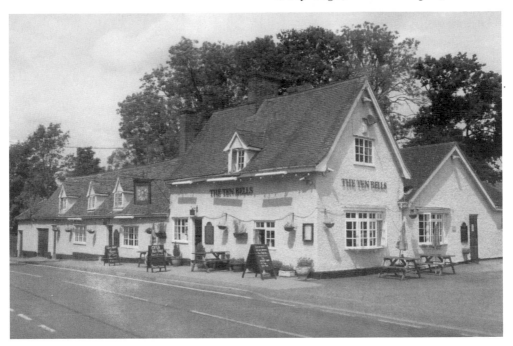

The Ten Bells, Stonham Aspal. (Author's collection)

but he was appalled at the state in which the family was living. James was lying in a very old bed with little in the way of coverings and there was no sign of either food or drink by his bedside. In fact it looked as if there was no food in the house at all. The following day James was dead.

The simple funeral was planned for Thursday. James's coffin was brought out of the house and the procession of mourners had already lined up ready for the journey to the church when the rector, the Revd Charles Shorting, arrived to declare that the ceremony could not take place until the messenger he had sent to Debenham had returned. The rector had become suspicious; he had heard rumours that the deceased's wife had recently purchased arsenic. In a small community it was not surprising that news of a death would spread quickly, but in this case it was soon known outside the village. The day after James's death, Elizabeth Lambert told her mother, who lived in Wetheringsett, about Mary asking her to buy poison. Gunn, the painter and glazier, heard about it from Mr Powell, the local solicitor in Debenham, in whose house he was working at the time. Both these sources recounted their meetings with Mary and each would have helped to spread the gossip. Alas, we are not told how long the procession was held up or what reaction there was from the chief mourner. But eventually the messenger, probably the rector's manservant, arrived with information that caused Mr Shorting to send details to E. Lawrence, the coroner, who ordered a post-mortem.

This was carried out by Mr Lock, assisted, as was customary, by another doctor. Neither had had much experience of post-mortems. Lock had examined the deceased's stomach and ilium and found they were perfectly healthy, as was the brain. In the stomach and small bowel he had found small particles of a mealy powder but no traces of arsenic. It is possible that Lock, who does not seem to have been over-scrupulous in keeping records of what he dispensed to his patients, was worried that his medicine might have contributed to the death because he stated categorically that he had not used arsenic in any of his prescriptions. However, the specimens were dispatched to forensic expert Mr Image at Bury St Edmunds for a more detailed analysis. He found arsenic and, interestingly, traces of vegetable matter which was identified as linseed meal. When questioned later, Mr Smith, who had sold the arsenic, described how for one penny he mixed six drachms of arsenic to an equal amount of linseed meal.

The inquest was held over three days; Friday, Saturday and Monday at the Ten Bells Inn. Mary had already been taken into custody awaiting the outcome of the inquest. It was serendipitous that the 1851 census should have been taken on 30 March. In their home in Stonham Aspal were listed son Richard under the heading of 'head of household', Sybilla and her baby daughter Jane, then a month old, William (fifteen), Betsey (nine) and Emma (seven) and brought in to look after them all was a friend, Rose Thurlow. John, then sixteen, was living-in at the farm where he worked. But the most interesting item from this census return was the one for neighbouring Little Stonham, where, in the house occupied by PC Whitehead and his wife Phoebe, was the entry for Mary Cage with the word 'prisoner' inscribed in the column reserved for 'relationship to the head of household'.

Mary did not stay there long. Once the inquest jury had brought in its verdict that 'James Cage died from poison administered by his wife', she was taken to the gaol in Bury St Edmunds to await trial at the next assizes. As luck would have it, when Mary was officially charged the Lent Assizes had opened the day before. The solicitor acting on her behalf asked for a postponement until the next assizes so that they could have time to prepare her defence. It would appear that suspicion had also fallen on Mary's son, James, but there must have been insufficient evidence against him for when the case came before Lord Chief Baron the Right Honourable Sir Frederick Pollock on 1 August, Mary alone was charged. Unlike Elizabeth Wooltorton (*see* Chapter One), whose fate was decided in three weeks from deed to death, Mary served four long months in Ipswich Gaol. She was, however, spared the journey back to Bury St Edmunds for the trial as the Suffolk Summer Assizes were held that year at the County Hall in Ipswich, which conveniently had the gaol situated behind it.

Detail from 1851 census for Little Stonham. (Author's collection)

The journalist who attended the trial on behalf of the *Ipswich Journal* took particular care to provide such details of the prisoner as he thought would catch the imagination of his readers. On trial for her life was a 'monstrous, heartless creature' who had murdered her husband, and yet was, he wrote, 'ordinary'. Not very tall, her dress covered by a faded coloured shawl and wearing a black bonnet, there was 'nothing repulsive in her countenance.' While the jury was being called, she stood motionless; her hands folded one over the other resting on the bar. Studying her closely, he noted that she had a somewhat drowsy look that, he suggested, indicated she was an opium eater. Whether he was right in this assumption we shall never know.

For most of us, opium smoking belongs to the realm of the Victorian poets and novelists who sought mystical experiences in back street dens in London, certainly not a habit to be found among the peasantry of Suffolk. Yet, according to an article in the *East Suffolk Gazette* and *Beccles and Bungay Weekly News*, opium eating was a huge problem throughout the eastern counties by the late 1860s. The article cited the case of a chemist in Kings Lynn who sold 200lbs a year of solid opium. Another sold 140lbs annually plus five to six gallons of laudanum and the same amount every week of the patent medicine Godfrey's Elixir, which had a pint of laudanum in every three gallons. The high incidence of drug-taking among the poor was blamed on the need to ease the pain they suffered, whether it be from near starvation, various feverish illnesses or an acute rheumatic condition common to most agricultural workers. Opium also contributed to the high infant mortality rate. The conclusion of the doctor responsible for the report was that the effects of opium eating on the rural population were far worse than syphilis.

The selection of the jury took a long time as Mr Gudgeon, one of the defence team, found reason to object to a number of them. The hold-up irritated the judge, who reminded him that an objection to twenty jurors was the limit. Finally, Mr Power, for the prosecution, was able to begin outlining the case. The press noted that Power gave a 'temperate speech'. He pointed out that the jury would have to consider the evidence that initially no arsenic had been found in the body, so had very small quantities been administered over a period of time in order to avoid detection? They should also bear in mind that during all the time James was ill at home, apart from Mary there had only been two other adults in the house during the day; Sybilla, the new mother, and son James, who was said to have once taken bread and butter to his 'stepfather'. (There is confusion here. Perhaps the reporter misheard or Mr Power used the wrong name, but later Richard in his evidence said *he* had taken the food to his father.) Only Mary had given the deceased medicine. Mr Power reminded the jury that if they were satisfied with the evidence they would hear then 'it was their bounden duty, however painful to say that the prisoner was guilty.' He went on to say that if his learned friend should 'satisfy them that any reasonable doubt existed, they would rejoice in giving their verdict in favour of her.' At this point Mary appeared to be about to faint, so she was allowed to be seated for the rest of the hearing.

Then followed all the evidence from the various witnesses including Mr Image, who stated that he had found arsenious acid in various tissues and traces of arsenic in the deceased's liver. He did not believe that the arsenic had been delivered in one dose. It was also his opinion, based on his analysis of the bodily specimens, that the amount ingested must have caused death. The prosecution called Mary Ann Betts, the daughter for whom Mary had persuaded Elizabeth Lambert to purchase rat poison. As Mrs Betts entered the witness box she looked as if she was about to faint. Despite being overcome by the solemnity of the occasion or by fear, she was able to find the words to firmly deny that she had ever had a rodent infestation.

The defence did its best to show that James Cage had a violent temper and his time in prison for beating up his wife was revealed to the jury. Mary's son Richard related that he had recently returned home to live after an absence of three years, and in his mother's defence he testified she had always been attentive and affectionate towards his father. However, under cross-examination he was forced to blacken Mary's reputation by admitting that she had twice left James, once with Robert Tricker.

In his summing up, counsel for the defendant, Mr Cooper, reminded the jury that the issue before them involved the life or death of the prisoner and he urged them to rid their minds of prejudice. Having heard all the evidence, paramount among the questions they needed to ask themselves was how had the deceased come by the poison? Had it been administered by Mary? He dismissed the evidence offered by Gunn about Mary saying she would soon find a new husband. Gunn was a great joker and Mary may well have answered in a joking way, as one often did when upset and under stress. Similarly, he poured doubt on the veracity of Elizabeth Lambert's version of events. How much had she added to her story after the arrest of the prisoner? Were they really expected to believe that the prisoner would so blatantly ask Lambert to procure poison for her if she was intending to kill her husband with it? And why was it that not a trace of arsenic had been found in the Cages' home when it was first searched by the police? Evidence had been given that Mary had stood by while the police constables had examined drawers and, when a paper package was found, Mary had said she'd been looking for it. This however contained not arsenic but the spice turmeric, used to stem the flow of blood from a cut.

So, continued Mr Cooper, could the deceased have taken the arsenic himself by mistake? He reminded the jury that Mr Lock, the medical practitioner, 'could not recall' if he had sent medication for James in liquid, pill or powder form. And was it not strange that the doctor had no suspicion at all that his patient was slowly and deliberately being poisoned but had continued to treat him for rheumatism?

It was then the turn of the judge to sum up. He reminded the jury that Mary stood charged with one of the few remaining charges which affected the life of the prisoner. If she was guilty then she must not be allowed to escape. At this point, Mr Cooper begged his Lordship's pardon to ask if his Lordship would enquire if Mary could read or write. Richard Cage was called back to testify that he knew she could not. Nothing further was made of the question but doubt over mix-ups of paper packages had been raised. The Chief Baron took an hour and a half to complete his summing up, during which time Mary sat with her body bent forward, her forehead in her hands. The jury was out for twenty-two minutes. According to the *Ipswich Journal*, there was 'a breathless expectation' in the crowded courtroom. The verdict was 'Guilty'.

Directing his remarks to Mary, the judge commented on the enormity of her crime, pointing out that she had been willing to walk four miles in order to procure poison. He also made general remarks about the number of poisoning cases that had come before the courts in recent years that had been committed by women. He then addressed Mary, saying:

> I can hold out to you no hope of mercy. It is impossible to suggest any consideration that can lead to any alteration of the sentence which it is now my unhappy duty to pronounce. I earnestly recommend and implore you, therefore, to direct your attention and employ your time in those religious exercises that befit your unhappy condition and the great and awful change which you must undergo.

The courtroom reporter noted that the sentence to be hanged by the neck was then passed in the usual form. He also noted that it seemed to him that his Lordship added the words, 'And may the Lord God Almighty have mercy on your soul' with great emphasis and deep feeling. Mary, who had remained seated throughout, now rose from her chair apparently in a very weak state and was helped from the dock. She was not, however, the only one to have been affected by the case; it was reported that at the end of the proceedings, Sir Frederick Pollock appeared to be 'entirely overcome' by his emotions and had left the court for a few minutes.

It was six years since Mary Sheming had been hanged in Ipswich, so the forthcoming event excited much public attention. The debate over the justification of hanging as a punishment was intensifying and, as the Catharine Foster case had shown, there was an even greater repugnance to the sight of a woman hanging from the end of a rope.

The execution was set for Saturday 19 August, two weeks after the end of the trial. As we know from other cases, this date could be altered, especially if a petition had been presented to the Queen begging for leniency towards the prisoner. It had already been indicated that this could not happen in Mary's case but her execution was in fact delayed for two days, for the very mundane reason that the hangman was not free to carry it out on the date specified. The famous executioner, William Calcraft from Newgate, was booked to officiate. Unfortunately he was already engaged on similar business in Norwich. The authorities tried as far afield as Gloucester for a deputy but none was found, so Mary had two extra days of life, though fortunately she had not been told in advance on which day her life would end.

In the two weeks left to her, Mary had plenty of chance to do as the judge had wished and employ herself in religious exercises. When taken back to the gaol following the trial, she had to pass through the gatehouse lodge, where she had a chance encounter with the prison chaplain, the Revd J.E. Daniels. He had taken one look at her and uttered, 'Come unto me all ye that are heavy laden and I will give you rest.' Mary had found great comfort in his words and so she was prepared to listen to everything the chaplain had to say to her over the next two weeks. He reported that her demeanour was marked by 'propriety, resignation and apparent penitence' as he tried to prepare her for her fate. She listened seriously to his advice and exhortations and declared her sorrow for the 'abandoned life' she had led. She expressed the hope that she might be permitted to obtain the means of grace.

However, in all their talks she steadfastly denied that she had committed the crime of which she was accused. The vicar of Stonham Aspal, the Revd Shorting, wrote to her offering words of comfort and begging her to make her peace by making a full confession. The letter was read to her by the chaplain, and she asked him to write her reply to Shorting. She told him the accusations against her were untrue and she had no idea who the murderer was. In reference to repenting for her sin, she replied, 'I have repented all I can bring to mind.' All in all, Mary impressed the chaplain. He thought she had great strength of mind and, although somewhat reserved and taciturn, she was sincere in her appreciation of his ministrations. She opened up to him about her past, telling him for example that she had once been so desperate she had contemplated committing suicide by throwing herself in a pond. Something, she knew not what, had held her back, and instead she had left her husband.

On the Thursday before her execution, Mary had a final meeting with most of her family. Richard, Mary Ann, Sybilla, William, Betsy and Emma came with her old friends Rose and Caroline Thurlow to say goodbye. Missing from the party were James and John. Mary gave each of her children a Bible, Testament, and prayer book in which the chaplain had written their names. Presumably this gift from Mary was financed by the chaplain. Relating that this visit took place, the *Ipswich Journal* reporter told his readers, 'they were all much overcome with the trying scene.'

On Monday evening, the Revd Daniels, joined by the Revd E. Bolton of Bramford, spent several hours keeping Mary occupied in religious exercises and prayer. They then left her to sleep, which she did for five hours. The chaplain then spent another hour with her between six and seven in the morning. He found her lying on her bed, very weak. She had not eaten breakfast and had in fact eaten very little since her conviction. He returned at eight thirty and remained with her until she was called from her cell. She told Daniels she was not afraid to die and thanked him for all he had done for her. She reminded him of his greeting to her on her arrival in the gaol and told him they would be the last words she would utter. She also thanked Mrs Johnson, the matron and wife of the prison governor for all her kindness. And then she was ready.

By 8.30 that Tuesday morning at least 500 people had gathered in St Helen's Street outside the gaol. The scaffold was ready. It had taken from just after ten o'clock on Monday evening until four o'clock that morning to erect it. There was a railing around it covered with black drapery to a height of 5ft, so as to leave only the drop visible. This arrangement was intended to conceal the appearance of the prisoner from the crowd until the last moment, but it was also calculated to add to the sombre and repulsive look of the structure. On that day the ghastliness of the instrument of death was particularly emphasised by the extreme brightness and freshness of a lovely summer's morning.

Detachments of both the County and Borough Police were lined up ready to preserve order. It being the time when labourers took their breakfast, many of them joined the stream of women and children who poured along the thoroughfares leading to the execution place. By nine o'clock the crowd formed a dense mass, filling the crescent-shaped space immediately in front of the gaol and extending back the whole length of Orchard Street through to Woodbridge Road. The roads to the right and left, up to the Dove Inn one way and to the corner of Upper Orwell Street the other, were occupied by latecomers. In the main the spectators were working folk; very few respectably dressed people were spotted among them. The occupants of surrounding houses had drawn their blinds or shuttered their windows against the sight.

The tolling of the funeral knell from the bell tower of nearby St Margaret's Church signalled the time had come. The gaol door opened. Mary, led by the chaplain and supported by two wardresses, followed by Mr Johnson the prison governor, and Mr J. Gooding the Under-Sheriff, moved slowly across the courtyard towards the entrance lodge. Calcraft, the executioner, met the procession and took his place at the rear. When they reached the lodge Mary's arms were corded and, at her request, a handkerchief was fastened over her eyes so that she might not see the scaffold. The prison turnkey assisted her up the steps. It was only when she was almost on the platform that she became visible to the crowd. At her appearance an eerie silence fell upon those watching and waiting.

Calcraft was close behind her and spared no time in placing her in the correct position under the beam which carried the noose. His request to her to stand quite still was unnecessary; she did not move an inch. As he placed the rope around her neck, Calcraft heard her keep her promise to the chaplain as she murmured the words, 'Come unto me all ye that are heavy laden and I will give you rest.' In less than a minute the preliminaries were ready. The executioner descended the steps to take up his place beside the bolt that would open the drop. All that could be seen was Mary's solitary figure. The silence was so intense it was as if the crowd was holding its collective breath. Then the Under-Sheriff gave the signal, the bolt was drawn and Mary Cage ceased to exist.

At the moment of the drop some wag in the crowd started to sing a song about the gallows. He was roundly turned on and berated by those around him. But the tension was broken. The crowd dispersed quickly, without causing the police any trouble. Once the deed had been done, there was no desire to linger and see the body hanging there as a grim reminder of the result of evil doing. The corpse was left on view for the usual length of time before it was cut down and taken for burial in the precincts of the gaol, the last service the chaplain did for Mary.

In many of the cases of murder or manslaughter during the Victorian age, the accused who had protested their innocence in court finally admitted their guilt just before their execution. This may have been encouraged by the strong religious view of the time that only those who confessed their sins would be admitted into heaven otherwise they would be condemned to spend eternity in the fires of hell. Mary's story provides evidence of how hard the prison chaplains of the period worked to save the souls of the poor wretches awaiting execution. Subject to so much talking and sympathetic religious teaching, it is small wonder that prisoners would wish to rid themselves of their sins. But Mary went to her death claiming her innocence. She had repented for all the wrong-doing she could think of, but killing James Cage was not among them. So if she didn't feed him the arsenic, who did?

The year after Mary's execution, two of her sons, John (eighteen) and William (fifteen), were brought before the magistrates for burglary. The following year John was found guilty of rape and sentenced to be transported for fourteen years. On 3 January 1856, John was carried off to Western Australia in the prison ship *William Hammond*. Were they just a dysfunctional family or would things have been different if Mary had not been accused of murder?

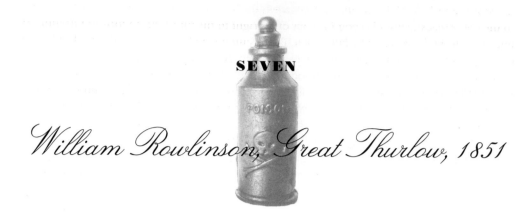

SEVEN

William Rowlinson, Great Thurlow, 1851

Those who resort to poison as a method of murder are not only spurred on by different motives, but can also be of varying ages. In this book, we have Catherine Foster (*see* Chapter Five) who was seventeen when she murdered her husband, while at the other end of the scale is seventy-eight-year-old William Rowlinson. What on earth, we may wonder, can possibly have driven a man – described in the press as a 'miserable old man' – to even contemplate murder? The answer, it would seem, was fear, jealousy and greed.

It was the year 1851 – an auspicious one in the history of Britain as the year of the Great Exhibition – but surprisingly, in Suffolk, it was also the year of a number of murders and murderous attempts.

William Rowlinson lived about a mile and a half out of Great Thurlow, on the way to Stradishall. The hamlet known as Sowley Green was then, as it is now, not much more than a farm or two and a handful of cottages with a drainage ditch forming the boundary with the lane. Today, the hamlet lies in the shadow of HM Prisons Highpoint and St Edmunds Hill. William lived next door to his son, another William, who was married with five children and until October 1850, he had shared the home of his other son, George, and his wife Mary. His working life had been spent as an agricultural labourer, but when he had become too frail to work a full day, he had been forced to seek Parish Relief. However, when he could, he supplemented his income by selling the dung he collected off the road. A bit of a miser, his needs must have been simple because he had managed to somehow accrue the sum of £11 5s and three farthings, a considerable sum in those days, especially for one on parochial benefit – benefit he would most certainly not have received had the Overseers of the Poor been aware either of such wealth or of the fact that he also owned a gold watch.

Sadly, in October 1850, William's son George died, leaving his few possessions to his wife. These included certain items of furniture that William thought he should have – possibly they had been passed down through his family. Initially, William was not unduly worried, until June of the following year, when Thomas Jermyn began courting forty-one-year-old Mary. The widow encouraged his attentions and eventually it was agreed that they would be married at Michaelmas, exactly a year to the day after George's death. Her father-in-law was very upset at the news, for it meant that Mary would be moving to live with Mr Jermyn – and that would mean Rowlinson having to find new lodgings. The outlook was bleak; his son William had no room for him, so either he had to find someone willing to take him in or submit to going into the workhouse. Mary's forthcoming marriage must have festered away inside him, and, added to the belief that she was cheating him out of his right to the furniture, he took the decision to put a stop to both problems by killing her. The decision may have been a rash one, but he was cunning enough to try and cover his tracks by slowly poisoning her to death.

Arsenic was, of course, his chosen poison. Benjamin White, the owner of the general stores in Great Thurlow, had no reason to believe that Rowlinson, whom he had known for over twenty years, was not telling the truth when he asked for poison to deal with an infestation of rodents at home, as he had done many times before and so he sold him the usual small amount. As Mr White was later to find out to his cost, he had failed to comply with the requirements of the new legislation brought in following the recent Act of Parliament of 5 June 1851 regarding the sale of arsenic. The legislators had thought of every contingency; the opening paragraph ended with details of procedure in the case of a purchaser unable to write (which was a large percentage of the population), with the injunction that the seller must add the words 'cannot write' against the name and further what should be done should a witness to the purchase be necessary. Mr White, as he had always done in the past, had simply written 'poison' on the small packet, and thought no more about the sale.

Following Mary's announcement of her forthcoming marriage, Rowlinson became very sullen and withdrawn, often acting in a petty manner. For example, on one occasion, when Mary came home at nine o'clock after having had tea with Jermyn and his family, she found that Rowlinson had locked the door and gone to bed. Unable to rouse him, she had been forced to spend the night at a neighbour's house. He had also taken to either providing his own food or eating meals wherever he could find them outside the house. Thus he was able to introduce arsenic into Mary's flour supply without endangering himself. As was usual, the flour for immediate use was kept in a large wooden box or trough on a stand. Mary's was a rough affair made of elm with an ill-fitting lid so it was never locked. Rowlinson kept his own bag of flour separate on the other side of the 'keeping room'.

His first attempt on her life took place on 7 August when, after using the flour to make herself a dumpling, Mary was violently sick. She recovered quickly and thought that she, like some of her neighbours, had a touch of whatever infection was going round at the time. A week later, in preparation for a visit from her sixteen-year-old niece Susan Cornell, Mary made a large blackcurrant pudding. Unfortunately, almost immediately after having eaten some of it both of them were taken ill. That the food might be responsible for their sickness never seemed to cross their minds. In fact when Susan went home, she took some of the pudding with her as a treat for the rest of her family. Her father Samuel and some of the younger members of the family ate it, but later they were all sick, each complaining that they felt a burning sensation in their throats before they vomited. Mr Cornell could not be sure that there was any connection with the sickness, but for some time after the event he experienced a strange numbness in his hands and feet.

Mary, meanwhile, was ill on and off throughout August. Since her widowhood she too had been receiving Parish Relief, mainly in the form of a bread allowance, but she was also entitled to seek the medical attention of the doctor employed under the Poor Law at the Union Workhouse. However, before she could see the doctor, Mr Baker, she had to visit the Relieving Officer to obtain the requisite order for medical treatment. She did not actually see Mr Baker on the first occasion but he dispensed medicine for her. At the time at least twenty-four of Mary's neighbours in Sowley Green were suffering from sickness and diarrhoea, so he assumed her case was no different to theirs and prescribed a purgative to clear the system.

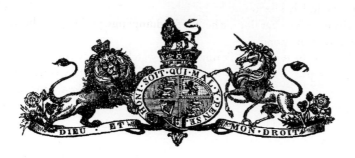

ANNO DECIMO QUARTO

VICTORIÆ REGINÆ.

****

C A P. XIII.

An Act to regulate the Sale of Arsenic.
[5th *June* 1851.]

WHEREAS the unrestricted Sale of Arsenic facilitates the Commission of Crime: Be it enacted by the Queen's most Excellent Majesty, by and with the Advice and Consent of the Lords Spiritual and Temporal, and Commons, in this present Parliament assembled, and by the Authority of the same, as follows:

I. Every Person who shall sell any Arsenic shall forthwith, and before the Delivery of such Arsenic to the Purchaser, enter or cause to be entered in a fair and regular Manner, in a Book or Books to be kept by such Person for that Purpose, in the Form set forth in the Schedule to this Act, or to the like Effect, a Statement of such Sale, with the Quantity of Arsenic so sold, and the Purpose for which such Arsenic is required or stated to be required, and the Day of the Month and Year of the Sale, and the Name, Place of Abode, and Condition or Occupation of the Purchaser, into all which Circumstances the Person selling such Arsenic is hereby required and authorized to inquire of the Purchaser before the Delivery to such Purchaser of the Arsenic sold, and such Entries shall in every Case be signed by the Person making the same, and shall also be signed

On every Sale of Arsenic, Particulars of Sale to be entered in a Book by the Seller in Form set forth in Schedule to this Act.

X x   by

The Act relating to sale of arsenic. (Reproduced by kind permission of OPSI)

He blamed this outbreak of English Cholera on their poor water supply drawn from the local pond. Possibly this would have been safe had it been boiled before use but Mary, like all the other housewives, always mixed her flour, whether for dumplings, puddings or bread, with cold water drawn straight from the pond.

Who can say what was in Rowlinson's mind as he watched Mary suffering the ill effects of the arsenic. However, just as he was about to renew his efforts, Mary offered lodging to a young single mother named Charlotte Sparkes. She and her two children, Emma, aged eleven, and Walter seven, had just come out of Risbridge Union Workhouse at Haverhill. Although at that time most women preferred to cook for their own families as it allowed them to control their housekeeping budgets, Mary had offered to provide them with board as well as lodging. To welcome the family on the day of their arrival Mary made them a seed cake. Rowlinson had sufficient conscience to try to warn Charlotte. Encountering her in the garden he advised her not to let her children eat any of Mary's food, telling her that it would make them ill, as she was such a very poor cook. That, he said, was why he never ate anything made by her. So Charlotte decided to keep her own supplies.

Towards the end of August, a week after the Sparkes had moved in, Mary was feeling so ill with stomach pains that between eight and nine o'clock one Saturday morning, she set out to walk the three miles to Wickhambrook to see Dr Stutter. Following an examination he gave her leeches to apply to her side. Realising that she would need assistance in applying them, when she got back home at half past twelve she sent for her sister, Ann Cornell, to come and help her. Later in the day, when a travelling salesman called, she bought a small piece of mutton from him to use as the basis for a broth which she hoped would do her good. Mrs Cornell arrived later that evening with her two youngest children.

The following day Mrs Cornell made dumplings to go with the mutton for dinner. Mary managed a little of the broth, as did the children, but Ann ate only the dumplings. It was not long before she was seized with violent stomach pains followed by continuous purging. She felt so ill that she wanted nothing except to be in her own home, but there was no way that she and the children could make the journey on foot back to nearby Barnardiston. So Mary sent her fiancé, Mr Jermyn, to fetch Ann's husband, who came with a cart in which to carry her home. He realised that she needed urgent medical attention but before he could send for the doctor he had to make a journey of six miles to obtain the necessary order from the Relieving Officer. It was therefore six o'clock when they eventually arrived home. Ann was put straight to bed and Mary Phillips, a neighbour, came in to help nurse her. In between her severe bouts of vomiting, she complained of intense thirst. Within two hours she was dead. Aged forty-five, she left ten children, the youngest of whom was just four years old.

Mr Baker, who had failed to reach Ann before her death, conducted a post-mortem the following day in the presence of Mrs Phillips. He opened up the body and removed the stomach, which he found to contain between a pint and a pint and a half of fluid. This he emptied into a basin and when he had replaced the stomach and sewn up the body he instructed Mrs Phillips to throw the fluid away. He felt there was no need for a more thorough examination as from the symptoms that had been described to him he assumed that the cause of death was English Cholera. At the inquest his declaration was accepted without question.

The enormity of what he had done in causing the death of Ann Cornell does not seem to have worried Rowlinson who, if anything, now became even more determined to be rid of Mary. At the end of harvesting, Mary joined other women in the fields to glean those ears of corn which had escaped from the sheaves of wheat and barley when they were bound up. With

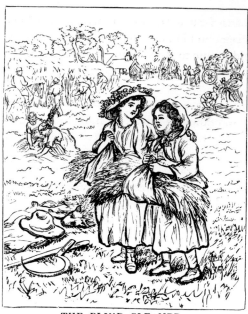

The Gleaners, taken from The Infant's Magazine, *1877. (Author's collection)*

THE BLIND GLEANER.

luck she would pick up enough grain to feed her chickens throughout the winter. It being the practice to take something to eat in the field during the midday break rather than returning home, Mary took a cold apple dumpling she had made earlier. After eating, she felt so ill with stomach cramps that she was forced to lie down among the stubble. She also experienced what she described as a burning thirst. On the previous day, when she had made her apple dumplings, Mary had taken some as a gift to her future mother-in-law. She was to discover later that when Mrs Jermyn had served them up to her family, they too had been ill. Still no one considered the food to be causing the problem.

The 2nd of October must have been a Monday, for Mary and Charlotte spent the morning together doing the washing. In the kitchen afterwards they both made dumplings for dinner. Mary made four and Charlotte, using her own flour, made three, one each for her and the children. The children were hungry that day for they ate all three of Charlotte's dumplings between them so Mary offered to share hers with Charlotte. They ate three of Mary's four. Rowlinson, perhaps getting impatient, must have upped the dosage of arsenic he had mixed into the flour because the effect on Mary and Charlotte was almost instantaneous. The children, who showed no signs of sickness, ran next door to seek help for the two women. It is not clear who decided to dispose of Mary's fourth dumpling but it was a fortuitous move. The dumpling was broken into pieces and thrown out into the yard for the cat and the dog. When they too became ill, Mr Baker, who had been called out to attend Mary and Charlotte, could not blame the English Cholera this time. Sensibly, he collected up the scraps the animals had left, plus specimens of their regurgitation, and with samples of the flour found in the house he sent them all for analysis.

Thus was set in motion the investigations which led to Rowlinson being brought first on the Wednesday before the Revd Mayd, the local magistrate, at the Crown Inn. When the old man admitted that he had purchased arsenic, he was ordered to be held on remand at the police station at Clare, where, it was reported, he did not eat for two days. On the Saturday Mr White, the shopkeeper, was called to the office of the magistrates in Haverhill, and questioned about his part in the affair. When he agreed he had sold arsenic to Rowlinson, he was informed he would be investigated further and in December he was charged with selling arsenic 'without complying with the form of the Act of Parliament.'

It was not long before the connection was made between the attempt on Mary's life and the 'mysterious death' of Ann Cornell. Her body was exhumed and a post-mortem conducted by Mr Baker. At the ensuing inquest the coroner ordered that Mr W.G. Stutter should arrange for further investigations. The next step was for Rowlinson to be brought before the six local magistrates. At the court, held in Clare police station, he was officially charged on the two counts: the murder of Ann Cornell and the attempted murder of Mary by administering arsenic. Rowlinson cut a pathetic figure and the magistrates were moved to allow him to sit at their table. It was reported that as the lengthy evidence against him was unfolded, he spent most of the time with his head upon the table, apparently overcome with emotion. At the end of the hearing he was again remanded and sent to Bury Gaol to await trial at the next assizes.

Rowlinson's case was heard at the Lent Assizes at Bury St Edmunds on 25 March 1852, immediately following that of William Baldry (*see* Chapter Eight). After several months in Bury Gaol awaiting trial, Rowlinson had deteriorated even further. His voice trembled as he pleaded not guilty and again he was allowed a chair in the dock. Much was made of his extreme age and decrepitude, it being noted that he was well past man's allotted span of three score years and ten. There was little new evidence given beyond the detailed analysis of the organs removed from Ann Cornell's body. Ironically, although Ann's body had started to decompose, her internal organs were found to be in good shape. Thanks to Baker's mishandling, the stomach contents

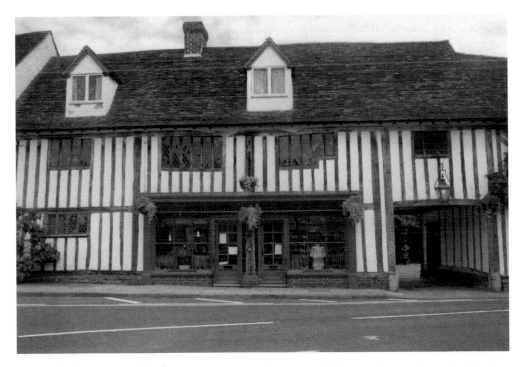

A house in Clare. (Author's collection)

had been lost, but there was sufficient mucous in the intestines to prove the presence of arsenic – the very poison which had helped to preserve the internal organs.

Mr Image stated the effects that arsenic poisoning had on a victim. These included vomiting and diarrhoea, thirst, sweating, collapse, nervous trembling, possible paralysis and inflammation of the eyes, feet and hands. In addition there might be swelling in different parts of the body as well as numbness of the feet and legs, making walking difficult. As Mary recounted her evidence, she was able to show that she had suffered from most of these symptoms and indeed Ann Cornell's widower still suffered from leg problems as a result of eating Mary's blackcurrant pudding months earlier.

The trial had started at 9 a.m. At one o'clock the governor of the gaol, who accompanied Rowlinson, indicated that the prisoner wished to leave the court. An adjournment of five minutes was allowed. The newspaper reported later that the prisoner was 'conducted from the Bar and seemed deeply depressed.' One assumes that it would have been indelicate to write in the newspaper that the prisoner wished to go to the lavatory. After sitting for four hours we might suppose that he was not the only one. There was no indication that there was any other recess during the course of the trial. When it resumed, Mr Power, for the defence, tried to suggest that the arsenic might have been accidentally scattered into the flour.

In summing up, the judge commented on the difficulty with trials such as this. He told the court:

> … with regard to poisoning, it is a crime of the deepest dye, one that it is hardly possible to bring home. It is a crime that is always committed in secret and it is only by circumstantial evidence that it can be brought home to the party accused.

As others had done during the trial, he drew attention to the laxity of the shopkeeper, who had sold arsenic as indifferently as if it had been 'merely sugarplums'.

At 3.15 p.m. the jury were invited to reach their verdict. However, they obviously felt the case was not cut and dried for they asked for permission to retire. They deliberated for almost an hour and three quarters before returning to give a verdict of guilty on both charges, but with a strong recommendation for mercy because of the prisoner's age and ill-health. The judge passed the death sentence but noted the jury's plea for mercy.

The date for execution was set. However, numerous petitions were sent to the Secretary of State begging for leniency on the grounds of Rowlinson's age and infirmity. It was hoped that his sentence would be commuted either to transportation or life imprisonment.

In the period following his sentence, it was reported that Rowlinson had confessed his guilt to a fellow prisoner but that he steadfastly refused to make the official confession to either the prison governor or the chaplain. Eventually, after another date was set for early May, word came that he was to be detained in gaol at 'Her Majesty's pleasure'. It was apparent to the authorities that this would not be for long as he was, in any case, now permanently bedridden in the infirmary and indeed his death followed not long after.

One must ask why, when a decision was usually reached in half an hour or so, the jury deliberated as long as they did in this particular case. Were they swayed by the pathetic figure that Rowlinson cut? Rowlinson's crime was in some ways similar to that of Elizabeth Wooltorton (*see* Chapter One), for both accidentally killed the wrong person. One could argue that Rowlinson was much more devious and determined than Elizabeth, yet her jury had no hesitation in condemning *her* to death.

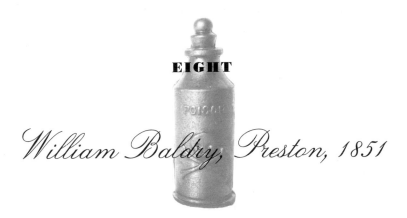

EIGHT

William Baldry, Preston, 1851

Most of those who appear in these accounts are drawn from the poorest level of society; those whose lives were especially hard, who lived in the meanest surroundings, knowing little of even the most basic of comforts. Lack of money was common to them all. Yet this particular case caused a frisson of shock around the county, for William Baldry was a member of the middle classes. It is interesting to note the courteous tone of the newspaper report of his appearance before the magistrate. The *Ipswich Journal* opted for the unsensational headline 'Case of Poisoning at Preston', followed by the comment, 'considerable excitement has been occasioned at Preston by a charge of attempting poisoning having been preferred against a respectable farmer. The party alleged to be implicated is Mr William Baldry.'

In 1851 William and Mary Baldry had been married for ten years. William was then thirty-four and Mary twenty-eight. Unusually for the time, they had only the one child, a one year-old son named James. Unfortunately, soon after his birth, the child had been diagnosed as 'an idiot'. The lack of previous children may be explained by the fact that Mary had suffered with ill health for a number of years. By her own admission she was of a 'nervous disposition', a condition which seems to have affected many women in those days. Although she consulted a number of doctors over the years, it would be wrong to dismiss her as a hypochondriac. She had been diagnosed as suffering from uterine irritability, known to cause either the inability to conceive or frequent miscarriages. The condition produced symptoms of unexplained vomiting as well as hysteria, which here is used in its original sense of irrational behaviour brought on by disturbance of the womb.

So Mary was frequently confined to her bed – a bed from which William was then excluded. However, it appears that he had been a most sympathetic and understanding husband, paying attention to her every need or whim. Then, in 1850, Mary had finally been able to carry a baby for the full term and, much to everyone's surprise, she had been extremely well throughout the pregnancy.

Outsiders can never gauge the true state of a marriage but the one problem that was known to exist between Mary and William was his shortage of money. William farmed in the village of Preston, a couple of miles from Lavenham – the picturesque medieval centre of the woollen industry – and four from Bildeston. The larger towns of Hadleigh and Sudbury were some nine miles distant. William came from farming stock but his own holding was not large as he only employed two labourers. From later evidence we learn that he raised pigs as well as crops.

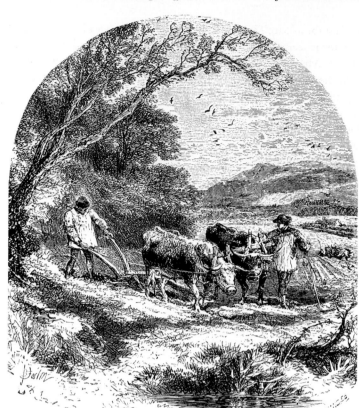

Ploughing. Taken from The Infant's Magazine, *1877. (Author's collection)*

Mary also came from a farming background. When her father died, his widow, Harriet Cone, took over the running of their farm with her son-in-law Leman Juby who, with his wife Susannah and their four children, lived with Harriet in the farmhouse at Whatfield. This was a much larger property than William's, consisting of 244 acres and employing seven men and three boys. The Cones' neighbours were the local rector and his family. Mary's father, James Cone, was sufficiently wealthy enough to pay Mary's medical bills, even though she was married, and he set up a trust fund to continue such provision for her after his death. On Mary's twenty-fifth birthday she had received from the trustees £350, a considerable sum when translated into today's money. Mr Cone had also specified that the money was to be solely for his daughter's personal use. The meant that it did not, as her other property did, pass automatically into the possession of her husband. Mary, however, generously gave William £100. It is not clear if she gave it out of sheer love for him and a desire to share her good fortune or if William expected – or even demanded – to have some of it. She herself apparently did not go on a wild spending spree, probably investing the rest, and two years after the initial gift, she gave William a further £50.

Then in the autumn of 1851, William asked for more. This time she refused to comply. He became very angry and, in Mary's mind, he thereafter seemed to be less kind and attentive. We have to ask why he needed the cash. The most obvious answer is that he was gambling and had got himself into serious debt. Had the farm been doing badly and he needed an injection of cash to buy stock or supplies it is likely that he could have borrowed from the bank or even asked his mother-in-law for a loan. Though whether Mrs Cone would have helped him is a matter for conjecture, for it seems clear that she was not particularly endeared to this son-in-law. It was the redoubtable Mrs Cone who became suspicious of his behaviour towards his wife and, had it not been for her quick thinking, she might well have lost her daughter.

Mary had been taken ill again in October. When she was unable to shake off a severe cold and sore throat, her mother came to stay to help nurse her. Mr Vincent, her medical practitioner, was in regular attendance too, as he had been for sometime before for her uterine problems. On this occasion the doctor was puzzled by the number of bilious episodes, which had such a debilitating affect on his patient. He had questioned her closely about her diet in an effort to find an answer there to her problem. It seemed strange to him that she should be seized with such violent vomiting after drinking a cup of tea or eating a bowl of nourishing pearl barley. He might have been alerted earlier had he questioned the maidservant, Sarah Hughes, and discovered that after she had mixed the remains of the pearl barley in with the poultry feed, several of the chickens and ducks had been found dead.

On the evening of 21 November, Mrs Cone came downstairs from Mary's room to make coffee. She poured out two cups, one for Mary and the other for William, then, realising that she had insufficient milk, she left the room for a minute or two to fetch some from the kitchen. On her return she sugared the coffee, gave William his cup and took the other upstairs to Mary. As she drank, Mary noticed a white sediment in the bottom of her cup. Somewhat fearfully, she poured the dregs into the saucer and gave it to her mother to examine. Mrs Cone was suspicious enough to decant some of these dregs into a small glass scent bottle. This she kept in her pocket to show to Mr Vincent on his next visit. She then bravely confronted William. Pointing to the sediment, she asked, 'What's this?' William's rather tame reply was that whatever

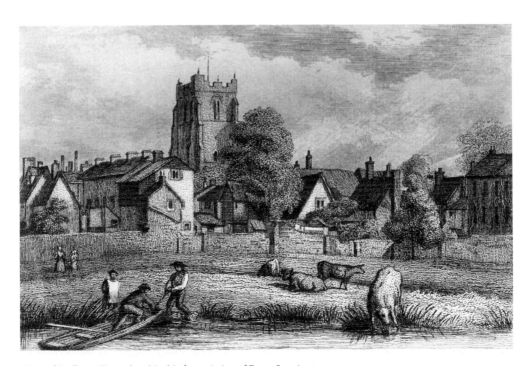

View of Sudbury. (Reproduced by kind permission of Roger Lane)

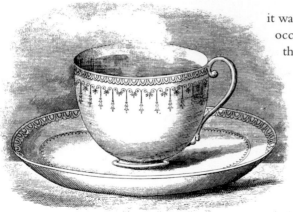

it was must have been in the sugar. On that occasion, although Mary felt unwell after the sips of coffee, she was not in fact sick.

A fortnight later, on 5 December, William paid his customary evening visit to his wife's bedside, this time bringing her a glass of beer. Mary did not want to drink it, saying Mr Vincent had forbidden her to have beer as she had been so ill on the last occasion her husband had given it to her. William persisted, saying it would help build up her strength. Mrs Cone grated a little nutmeg on the top and then watched as William stirred in a spoonful of sugar from a bowl that stood on the washstand. Mary remarked that her husband had stirred long enough and, taking the glass, she noted that the contents looked milky. Turning to her mother, she asked her if a clean glass had been used. Assured that it was, Mary reluctantly drank half the beer but was almost immediately sick and seized with stomach cramps.

In the early hours of the following morning, Mary was so seriously ill with the now familiar sickness and stomach pains, as well as a raging thirst, that Mrs Cone woke William to demand he send for the doctor immediately. After Mr Vincent had done what he could to ease Mary's plight, Mrs Cone showed him the phial of coffee dregs. He instantly identified the sediment as arsenic but said it must be sent to Mr Image for a thorough analysis. When he received Image's report, Vincent had enough evidence to take to the local police, and on 17 December he accompanied PC Payne to arrest William for attempted murder.

When confronted with the evidence against him, William confessed that he had purchased two powders from Mr Atwood of Bildeston because he felt he needed purging. There was a general belief at the time that if one were 'out of sorts' then a purging of the system – a bit like the modern detoxification – would improve ones health. He said he had taken one powder himself and had felt so much better after it that he thought it would help Mary. It was, of course, a recognised fact that doctor's prescriptions often contained small traces of arsenic.

In his panic, William tried to persuade both Mr Vincent and the police constable to say nothing about what had happened. He then implicated himself further by trying to bribe them. He took Vincent outside to the pigsty and showed him three fine, fat pigs and told him to choose one, while in the doctor's hearing he asked the policeman to name the price for his silence.

William was taken into custody and brought before the magistrate, the Revd N.W. Hallward, at Bury on 24 December. William was able to engage his own solicitor, Mr Goodhay, to represent him at the hearing. Mary was too ill to appear in court so her deposition was read for her. Mrs Cone gave her evidence, as did Mr Vincent about the phial containing the arsenic. And Sarah revealed for the first time what had happened to the ducks and chickens after eating the mistress's left-over pearl barley, thus indicating that William had been doctoring her food for longer than the two attempts with the beer and coffee. Sarah also confessed that she had treated herself to a cup of the left-over coffee and had suffered the vomiting and stomach pains now recognised as symptoms of arsenic poisoning. As his crimes were unravelled by the various witness statements, William sobbed loudly. The magistrates found him guilty of attempting to

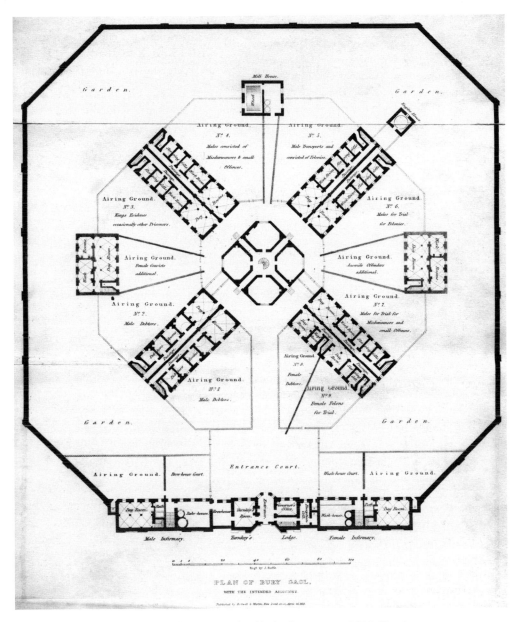

Plan of Bury Gaol. (Reproduced by kind permission of SRO/Bury)

administer poison with intent to destroy life and ordered him back to Bury Gaol to await the Lent Assizes.

William's trial took place on Thursday, 25 March 1852. When charged, he answered 'not guilty' in a firm tone. That Mary was still ill when she entered the witness box was apparent for all to see and the judge requested that she be seated to give her evidence. She added little to what she had said in her previous statement. Interest lay much more in what the various medical men had to say. Vincent outlined Mary's medical problems and gave details of the tests that had been carried out on the phial containing the coffee dregs. He, and later Mr Image, the expert witness, reported that there was no doubt that the white sediment was arsenic. According to William, he had bought the two powders from Mr Atwood for his own use. Atwood, who had been brought down from Camberwell where he now practised, told the court that he had at one time lived in Bildeston and had attended Mary between April and July 1847, but denied emphatically that he had ever sold any powders or poisonous matter of any description to William.

The defence argued that William had not premeditated the attempt on his wife's life and in fact tried to suggest that Mary's mother, Mrs Cone, might have been responsible for the poison appearing in both the coffee and the beer. The only evidence the lawyer could produce for this theory was to question why she had waited so long before handing the phial containing the coffee dregs to Mr Vincent. The case concluded at 8 p.m., at which point the court was adjourned, the judge directing that the members of the jury should be accommodated at one of the inns in the town under the supervision of a Sheriff's officer.

When the court opened the next day, Friday, William, who had had a night to consider his fate, was described as wearing an anxious and careworn look. He stood, his head hanging down, his hands grasping the front of the dock. The judge reminded the jury that the prisoner had been indicted for the offence of having administered poison to his wife with intent to kill. That was a capital offence so they must be absolutely certain as to his guilt. The jury asked leave to retire but it took them only a quarter of an hour to reach their verdict of guilty.

Placing the symbolic black cap on his head, the judge addressed the prisoner, saying that whatever his motive was, it was known only to God and his conscience. Then followed the traditional words: 'The sentence upon you is that you be taken from hence to the place from whence you came and from there to a place of execution and that you be there hanged by the neck until you be dead and,' – with great emphasis – 'may the Lord have mercy upon your soul.' At this, William raised his hand to his brow, burst into tears and slowly left the dock accompanied by two officers of the gaol.

And there the story might have ended except for a vivid newspaper report of the hanging, but it did not. On 3 April, the *Ipswich Journal* reported that a petition signed by a great number of people had been sent to Her Majesty's Secretary of State pleading that William's sentence be commuted to one of transportation. While a reply was awaited, William Baldry's execution was delayed until 8 May.

And what of Mary during this time? What thoughts went through her mind as her husband languished in gaol? Did she go to visit him? Or did her mother and friends try to persuade her to cut him right out of her life? While these speculations cannot be answered, what Mary actually did following her husband's sentence came as a surprise. Disregarding the general petitions, Mary sent one of her own directly to Queen Victoria, woman-to-woman, begging to have her husband's life spared. She said that had she realised that it would mean his death, she would never have been a party to his prosecution even though her own life had been at risk. His death, she believed, would hasten her own. It was with great reluctance that she had yielded to the solicitations of her friends to prosecute and only then was it in the certain belief that the extent of his punishment for his offence would be transportation or imprisonment. She begged Her Majesty to save her from the misery of knowing that she had destroyed her husband by having his sentence commuted to some less severe punishment that would spare his life.

On 1 May, the Clerk to the Assizes informed the *Ipswich Journal* that the judges had confirmed the sentence of death on William. On hearing the news, William himself promptly collapsed and was admitted to the prison infirmary. Readers of the newspaper were informed that the execution would now take place on 8 May. But when that day came, a last minute message was received from the Secretary of State. William was to be detained in prison at Her Majesty's pleasure. Perhaps Mary's petition had touched the royal heart. Or had the prison authorities conveyed to the Secretary of State that William's health was such that, as with Rowlinson, they need hardly go to the expense of an execution? The newspapers did not bother further with him, but sometime between May and August his death was registered.

Curiosity leads us to ask what happened to Mary next; how did she, an invalid with a severely handicapped child, manage? Surprisingly, the answer seems to be very well indeed. Within a year of William's death she married John Juby, several years her junior and the brother of her sister's husband. John had a large farm at Witnesham and it was there she and little James joined him in the latter part of 1853. Whatever gynaecological problems Mary may have experienced in the past did not prevent her from conceiving now, and her first daughter was born in 1854, to be followed by two sons and another daughter during the next five years. Mary was still living with her husband in 1901 when the death was recorded of her son James Baldry, who had remained throughout his life in the care of his mother and stepfather.

Had William been slowly poisoning Mary for years? Was he indeed responsible for turning her into an invalid? And did he then tire of the sickly wife who had added to his woes by producing a handicapped child? Did he hope to be rid of both? Or was it that his money problems were so pressing that he hoped to solve them by inheriting her money on her death? Like Elizabeth Wooltorton (*see* Chapter One), for the sake of a few hundred pounds, he lost everything.

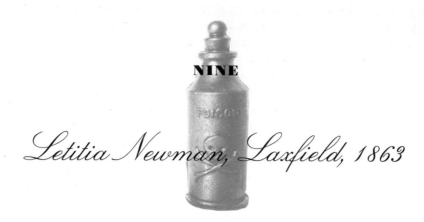

NINE

Letitia Newman, Laxfield, 1863

The old adage that hell hath no fury like a woman scorned may well provide the motive for Letitia Newman's attempt to murder William Keeble. Being spurned is bad enough for a young woman, but when one is forty-five and still a spinster, as Letitia was, then to see what may have been her last chance of marriage and financial security disappearing may have been more than she could bear.

The 1861 census for Stradbroke reveals Letitia as the head of a household, which consisted only of her and an elderly female lodger. Her occupation was given as charlady, but it was as a nurse that, in 1863, she entered Keeble's home in Badingham, a few miles away. He engaged her from the Tuesday after Whitsuntide to look after his seriously ill wife and when three weeks later, around 20 June, Rachel Keeble died at the age of thirty-eight, Letitia stayed on to act as housekeeper to the widower and to look after his four children.

It was not long before she was providing more than routine material comfort for the motherless family; she was also satisfying the physical needs of the bereaved husband. And in due course she suspected she was pregnant. We should not be surprised at the speed with which this happened or the possibility that she expected Keeble to marry her soon afterwards. In the early part of the nineteenth century, a working widower with children would waste no time in finding a new wife. In his 'Memoirs', Richard Stopher of Saxmundham recorded that he attended the funeral of a friend at which, by the end of the evening, the widower had proposed to another woman and plans were made for the marriage. Shakespeare too wrote of funeral-baked meats serving for the wedding feast in *Hamlet*.

However, Keeble, while happy to sleep with Letitia when it suited him, was not anxious to make the arrangement permanent. It appeared that when she told him she thought she was pregnant, the relationship became acrimonious. In one heated row he not only pushed and shoved her, he also slapped her face several times. He also suggested she take the powders he had procured that would produce an abortion, a charge he was to strenuously deny since it was illegal.

We know little about Keeble beyond the fact that he was by trade a sheep dresser and a butcher. The former occupation involved cleaning and preparing fleeces, a process in which arsenic was used in great quantities. Stored in the unlocked outhouse in his backyard during the thirteen-week period of Letitia's stay, Keeble had had at least a hundredweight (112lbs) or more of the poison packed in 4lb paper bags. By the end of August his stock had dwindled to between 30lb and 40lb. As far as the butchery was concerned, this probably means that he slaughtered and cut up the animals he supplied to others rather than running an actual butcher's shop as we know it. We know too that to pursue his trade he needed transport, so he owned a horse and cart, both of which he kept at the White Horse in Badingham.

Perhaps the only other relevant fact we need to know about him is that he obviously had a roving eye, as while he was 'leading on' Letitia, he was also courting another, younger woman by the name of Mary Ann Jenkins. When Letitia challenged him on this relationship, he decided she must go. So, reminding her of her position in the house, on 20 August he gave her a month's notice. However, on the morning of 2 September, long before the notice period had elapsed, Keeble applied to PC Larkin, who was stationed in the nearby village of Dennington, to come and be a witness that he was dismissing her instantly, as her conduct had become so bad. In the presence of the policeman, Keeble informed her she was legally discharged. Letitia tried to demand her rights and refused to leave. However, when the constable advised her to go quietly, she packed her belongings and left the house.

Still fuming when she stepped out onto the unpaved street, she picked up some old broken brick-ends and hurled them at the house, and when Keeble and the policeman emerged and walked to the White Horse – about a hundred yards down the road – she pelted him with stones, some of which met their target. While she was searching for further ammunition, a passing neighbour, Mrs Maria Lockwood, stopped and asked her what she was doing. Letitia said she had lost half a crown, a not inconsiderable sum in those days. Not finding it on the ground, Mrs Lockwood suggested she turn out her pocket to make certain the coin was not there. The pocket in question would have been a separate drawstring bag that was tied round the waist. Helpful Mrs Lockwood put her hand in and withdrew a little piece of twisted newspaper. Could the half crown have got inside there, wondered Mrs Lockwood. As she was about to unwrap it, Letitia took it from her, but not before Mrs Lockwood had had time to see that it contained some white powder. This, she assumed, was magnesia, commonly used to relieve indigestion. Letitia had put the powder back in her pocket and Mrs Lockwood went on her way, no doubt somewhat disgruntled that her help had been dismissed.

In the meantime, Keeble and PC Larkin were in the White Horse enjoying a quiet pint of porter, a strong, dark bitter beer. Their peace was shattered when Letitia entered the public house and began abusing Keeble for his treatment of her and saying that the least he could do was to drive her back to her home in Stradbroke. Keeble refused, saying, 'I don't know I have any right to send you home. You have money (he had settled her wages) and can pay your own way home.' However, the policeman advised Keeble to get his horse and cart and drive her on the grounds that she was a bad lot and 'the sooner she was gone the better.'

Letitia was indeed well known to the police in the locality. And she was no stranger either to Ipswich Gaol. Some change in her circumstances when she was twenty-three led to her going into the Hoxne Union Workhouse at Stradbroke as a pauper. Instead of accepting her lot with gratitude, Letitia refused repeatedly to work. She was reported to the authorities and ended up sentenced to one month's imprisonment with the addition of hard labour. The following year she was classed as a 'rogue and vagabond' and sentenced to three months hard labour. During the next ten years she was in and out of both the workhouse and prison, having set up a cycle of refusal to work in the Union workhouse and then being imprisoned. Her additional misdemeanours included disorderly behaviour and assault.

Had he known this, Keeble would no doubt have thought twice about employing her. Now, reluctantly, he took the policeman's advice and as he was going to Halesworth on business

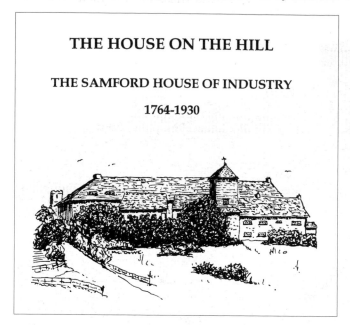

THE HOUSE ON THE HILL

THE SAMFORD HOUSE OF INDUSTRY

1764-1930

A Suffolk Union Workhouse.
Drawing by M. Dowe. (Author's
collection)

anyway, he agreed that he would take her as far as Laxfield. Since there is no indication of what conversation took place on that short journey, we can only assume that both parties had calmed down sufficiently so that when they alighted at the public house in Laxfield, another White Horse, they were on civil enough terms for them to enter the kitchen of the house which served as the public bar and to share a mug of porter. Assuming his position of superiority, Keeble drank at least half of it and then passed it to Letitia to finish while he went out to arrange with the landlady, Mrs Balls, about feed for his horse. While he was talking to Mrs Balls in her wash-house, he told her some of his story and confided that he did not wish to drive Letitia any further. Returning to the bar, Mrs Balls saw Letitia shake the mug of beer and then brush off what appeared to be a white dust that was scattered over the table with her handkerchief. When asked what she was doing, Letitia explained she had spilt some of the beer.

Mrs Balls immediately turned tail and went out to the stables to tell Keeble. When he returned to the table he picked up the mug and saw that there was white stuff floating on the top of the porter. This he immediately identified as arsenic. Holding the mug out, he told Letitia to drink it. She refused, saying, 'No, I durst not drink any more as it makes my head ache.' Keeble called to Mrs Balls to bring him a clean pint mug. Pouring the contents of the original mug into the clean one, a white sediment was left at the bottom of the first. Then he challenged Letitia, 'What made you put poison into this mug to destroy my life?' At which point, she jumped up, grabbed the second mug and threw the contents outside into the yard. When asked why she had done that, she replied, 'I couldn't drink it and you wouldn't.'

For the second time that day, Keeble sent for a policeman, this time to have Letitia charged with an attempt on his life. Mrs Balls removed the clean mug while Keeble kept the one with the dregs to hand over to the constable as supporting evidence.

PC Charles Hunt, who was stationed in the village of Laxfield, duly arrived and having heard statements, he cautioned Letitia. She was at that stage quite confident and more or less

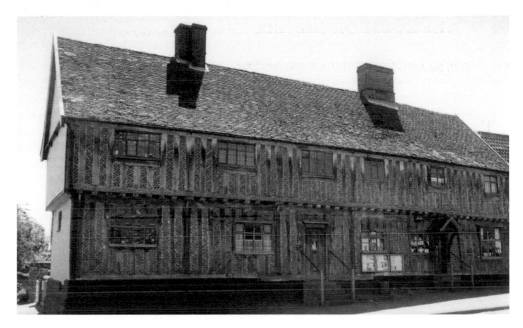

Laxfield Guildhall. (Author's collection)

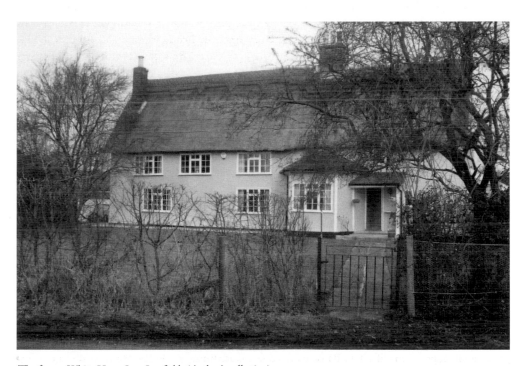

The former White Horse Inn, Laxfield. (Author's collection)

told him he could say and do as he liked, because there was not much he could do as no one had actually seen her put the arsenic in the porter. Nonetheless he arrested her on suspicion and took her and her accuser to the police station in Stradbroke. So she got her ride to that village after all, even though it was not to her home as she had hoped. The policeman also took charge of the mug containing the sediment to send to Mr Charles Read, the surgeon and apothecary at Stradbroke, for analysis.

Once she was in the police cell, Letitia had time to consider her situation. It may be that she hoped to persuade Keeble to drop the charge for she asked if she could speak to him. When the station sergeant told her he had gone, she said she realised she had done wrong and accepted that she was likely to have to go to prison.

The following day she was brought before the magistrates at Hoxne Petty Sessions charged with having 'attempted to cause to be taken by William Keeble, half a drachm of arsenic with intent to murder'. The most important witness was Mr Read, who testified that he had carried out various tests for arsenic, all of which had proved positive. The mug had contained between half a drachm and a drachm of arsenic, enough to destroy life. As a warning to anyone else who might consider repeating this crime, he pointed out that arsenic was not soluble in beer but becomes suspended in it, hence Letitia's attempt to shake up the porter. After she had been cautioned by the magistrates, Letitia said, 'I don't wish to make any statement, its no use saying anything now it is done.' She was remanded in Ipswich Gaol to await trial at the Lent Assizes.

In the nineteenth century it was unusual for a prisoner to have to wait long before being brought to full trial; a maximum of three months seems to have been the norm. But for some reason it was six months before Letitia was taken to Bury St Edmunds to appear at the Assizes, held in the last weeks in March. Her case was due to be heard on the 24th, a Thursday, but when the morning came there was no one present to represent the prisoner. After some discussion from the bench, the judge asked Letitia who her solicitor was. She replied that she did not know but that Mr Alloway, the governor of the gaol, would know his name. The judge then asked her when she had seen the solicitor. Learning that it had been the previous day in Ipswich Gaol, the judge asked her what he had said. She answered, 'He said he would do all he could for me.'

Having ascertained that Mr Mosely from Framlingham was the solicitor in question and that he was not present anywhere in the building, the prosecution solicitor suggested to the judge that a telegraphic message be sent to Mr Mosely to ascertain if he had indeed been retained to defend the prisoner. The judge commented on the laxity of Mr Mosely but agreed that the case should be held over to the following day.

On Friday morning the prosecution outlined the facts of the case. The only bit of excitement came when Keeble, in giving his account of events, said that when he accused Letitia of poisoning the beer she had said, 'You are a liar and no one haven't seen me do it.'

'I am not a liar, moreover this woman, Mrs Balls, saw you put it in,' he had replied.

'Then Mrs Balls is a liar likewise,' the prisoner had declared.

This was too much for Letitia, who shouted out from the dock, 'I never said no such thing.'

Perhaps because of his failure to appear the previous day, Mr Mosely tried to do his best for his client. During his cross-examination of Keeble, he questioned why it was, if he had been wary of the prisoner's temper, he had been quite happy to let her take on the management of his children and cook their meals? Mosely then went on to probe the close relationship which had developed between employer and employee, asking if the rows that they had were over Keeble's visits to the public house – and his interest in another woman. Without waiting for an answer the solicitor then raised the question of Letitia's 'certain condition'. Had she told Keeble of it? He agreed that she had but he could not remember when, only that she had gone on and on about it. He adamantly denied that he had ever given her either medicine or powders that would have altered her 'condition'.

Much having been made by the prosecution of Letitia's fiery temper, Mr Mosely now forced Keeble into admitting that he had frequently hit her. Asked if he had ever kicked her, he answered 'no,' but admitted that he might have pushed her. When asked how hard, he replied, 'hard as I could, though I was lame at the time so couldn't push too hard.' Continuing with this line of questioning, Mosely forced Keeble into admitting that the few stones and brick-ends that Letitia had thrown at him had not really hurt him at all. In fact, he even agreed that when the pair had driven off to Laxfield they were friends again.

There was a sharp intake of breath as Keeble admitted that since the episode in September he had remarried, followed by an outburst of laughter in court when in answer to the question 'Who to?' he replied, 'A woman.' But gravity was restored when he was asked how high off the ground his large stock of arsenic was kept. Would the jury question if 15ft seemed rather high for the average person to reach?

Mosely then recalled Mrs Balls for further questioning. Was it possible that the powder she had allegedly seen Letitia place in the mug might not have been magnesia? She agreed that she had heard of the practice in some public houses of adding soda to beer to give it a head, but her porter was good and did not need any addition. Summing up, Mr Mosely reiterated that Keeble, having taken advantage of Letitia, wanted to get rid of her when she became pregnant. That, with his abusive treatment, had exasperated her beyond endurance, hence the throwing of the brick-ends. She had, he believed, either put the powder in to the drink believing it was magnesia or, knowing it was arsenic, had intended to drink it herself but had faltered at the last minute.

Addressing the jury, the judge said that the prisoner was charged with 'intent to murder' so they must decide first did she know the powder was arsenic? Second, did she put it in the mug and third, if she did, was it with intent to murder? It was also their duty to consider if she might have intended to drink it herself while he was feeding the horse.

In spite of Mr Mosely's spirited defence and the judge indicating that there was room for doubt, the jury needed only a short time to consider before they returned their verdict of 'Guilty'. However, since the attempt on Keeble had failed, the death penalty was commuted to penal servitude for life.

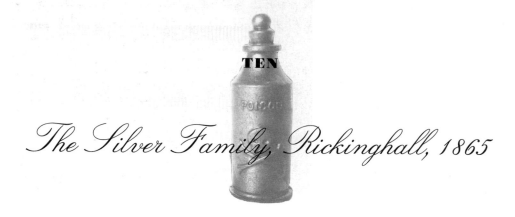

TEN

The Silver Family, Rickinghall, 1865

Not every case of poisoning by arsenic was a deliberate attempt to take another's life. There were some occasions when the poison was administered unwittingly and others when it was taken by accident. Time and again we read that it was commonplace for poison to be kept either in the house or an outbuilding to destroy vermin, or used as a basic ingredient in a preparation to treat animals. However, when a sudden death occurred following symptoms that might well be those now recognised as being of arsenic poisoning, then, as with all cases of sudden death, it became a matter for investigation by the local coroner.

The large village of Rickinghall Inferior, a suburb of Botesdale, lies close to Suffolk's border with Norfolk. Indeed the Church of St Mary, with its circular tower, shows the influence of the northern county rather than that of Suffolk. In the 1860s the local inhabitants were more likely to have visited the markets in Diss than other towns in the county, though the local carriers had a twice-weekly service to both Bury St Edmunds and Ipswich. Most of the men would have been employed on one of the eight farms and the presence of a resident veterinary surgeon suggests that animal husbandry was important there. There was also enough work to support two blacksmiths. The village had its own corn mill and, as well as the usual tradesmen and a couple of shops, it ran to a confectioner – not the mundane purveyor of boiled sweets – but a craftsman selling cakes, pies and tarts.

It was at the Bell Inn in Rickinghall Inferior on Saturday 5 August 1865 that J. W. Ion, the Deputy Coroner, held an inquest into the sudden death four days earlier of little Charley Silver. Charley, who was two and a half, had lived with his parents, Richard and Sophia, and three brothers in the last house in Water Lane, a home they had occupied for the past two years since Richard had taken up employment at one of the local farms. As its name suggests, the area was low lying and damp and Sophia was firmly convinced that it was an unhealthy location as none of the children had really been well since they moved there.

A picture of the family's life unfolded as evidence was given to the coroner. On the Sunday evening when they had gathered round the table for tea, little Charley had sat beside his father. Soon afterwards he and seven-year-old David went to bed, to be followed a short time later by Robert, who was nine. Around midnight, Charley became restless in the bed he shared with his parents, waking his father as well as his mother to say he did not feel well. Not long after, Isaac, who was five, complained to his mother that he had 'a sore head'. Robert was the first of the children to get up on Monday and had started on his usual breakfast of bread and butter

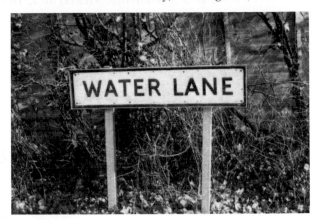

Road sign for Water Lane, Rickinghall.
(Author's collection)

when Charley came down. Robert sat up at the table but Charley took his slice of bread and sat down on the rug by the hearth. All the children had the same to eat, washed down by a mug of sugared tea, poured from the same pot as the one from which their mother also drank.

Before Charley had finished his meal, Robert left the house to take breakfast to his father in the fields. Knowing that he would return soon and keep an eye on Charley, Mrs Silver set out to walk to the doctor's surgery in Botesdale with Isaac, who was still suffering with a severe headache. Charley meanwhile played in the garden at the front of the cottage, where he was seen by their next-door neighbour, Mrs Elizabeth Spear, at around 7.30 a.m. as she was on her way to do a day's brewing. She stopped to speak to the child, who seemed perfectly all right to her. However, when she returned to have her breakfast at nine o'clock, she encountered Charley and Robert in the lane leading to Norton's farm. Charley was holding on to his brother's hand and crying. Mrs Spear asked what the matter was and was told he had been sick. Robert volunteered the information that when he had found Charley in Warner's field, he had already been sick and he continued to be so.

Mrs Silver arrived back home with Isaac at about ten o'clock to find that she now had two ailing children. Charley vomited throughout most of the day and his mother was at a loss what to give him beyond sips of cold tea. She made a makeshift bed out of pillows for him beside the kitchen fire so that he was under her constant supervision. But when there was no sign of improvement as the day wore on, she consulted Mrs Spear – an authority on childhood illnesses as her own children were often ill. Mrs Spear's first question was to ask if Charley had eaten something he should not. Mrs Silver said that as far as she was aware he had not. On her neighbour's advice, Mrs Silver visited the doctor again that evening for something that might stop the sickness and alleviate the obvious pain the child was in. It was eight thirty when she arrived at Mr Pearce's surgery. He had just been called out to attend a case and was in a hurry, so having listened, perhaps somewhat perfunctorily, to what she had to say, he gave her the standard medication for an upset stomach in the form of powders.

Bearing in mind that this was August, Richard Silver would have spent a very long and arduous day in the harvest fields. When he returned home hungry and tired and feeling the effects of having had his sleep disturbed the previous night, he went to bed as soon as he could, leaving his wife to deal with the sick child. During the night Sophia gave Charley one of the prescribed powders, which made him vomit almost immediately. Richard left for work at 4.30 a.m. on Tuesday morning, most likely unaware of the seriousness of his son's condition. Had he

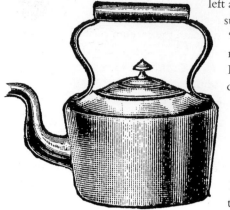

left a little later he would have been there to see Charley suddenly sit up in bed, his eyes rolling wildly, calling 'Mummy, Mummy'. Finally, at about half past five, not knowing what more she could do, Sophia sent Robert to ask another neighbour, Sarah Brock, to come and help her. Mrs Brock found the distraught mother sitting in the bed holding Charley to her. To Mrs Brock's practised eye, the child appeared to be suffering from convulsions. Sophia Silver was by now convinced that Charley was dying, telling Sarah, 'he is being taken just as the other was.' Mrs Brock did her best to comfort her but also made the practical suggestion that medical attention was needed. So off went young Robert again, this time to ask Mr Pearce to call as soon as he could.

Pearce arrived in under an hour and examined Charley, who was by then in a comatose state. The child was experiencing both breathing problems and violent muscle spasms throughout his body, but particularly in his legs. The surgeon felt the little boy's hands and found they were cold and moist, though his feet were warm. His barely perceptible pulse was rapid. Further examination revealed that his jaws were locked and his pupils fixed and dilated. The little lad's face and lips were a ghastly leaden blue colour, but what the surgeon found most worrying was the frothing at the mouth.

Mr Pearce recommended the standard procedures of the time. Mustard poultices were to be applied to Charley's abdomen and the calves of his legs, followed by a warm bath which would stimulate his heart and warm his extremities. In an effort to make his pupils contract he was to be placed near light. The two women busied themselves in carrying out these instructions and when Charley rallied for a time it looked as if they had been successful. But the improvement was only temporary. He relapsed to his former state and by two o'clock he was dead.

Twenty-first century readers may find Richard Silver's reaction to his son's death puzzling. To start with, when asked at the inquest if he was the father of the child, he said, 'I believe I am the father of Charley.' Was this simply a rather formal response to a formal occasion or did he have reason to doubt his paternity? And then he revealed that although he had been informed of Charley's death at half past three in the afternoon, he had not gone home until the usual time of seven thirty. Surely, no employer would have been so hard-hearted as to make a man work on in those circumstances? Indeed not. The choice had been Richard's; he 'did not see any occasion to go home for all that.'

Almost immediately after the death, gossip began to circulate that Charley had been poisoned. Sophia, still in a raw state, went on the Wednesday morning to ask Mr Pearce if he could find out what had caused her son's death. Pearce told her that it was violent inflammation of the chest. However, having considered the fact that the symptoms Sophia had described on Monday night certainly had not suggested that the case was so serious, and pondering on what he had seen during Charley's last hours and then learning that the Silvers had lost another child only a month before under similar circumstances, he decided a post-mortem was necessary. So on Wednesday afternoon he called again at the cottage in Water Lane to carry out his examination. At the same time he asked if the Silvers had any arsenic in the house. Sophia denied emphatically that she had ever had any.

Until such time as his funeral took place, Charley's little corpse was laid out in the cottage. And it was there, twenty-six hours after his death, that Pearce opened up the small body and removed the stomach, part of the small bowel, the rectum and the caecum of the large bowel, the pancreas and the spleen, the right kidney, the urinal bladder and its contents and the right lung. These items were carefully placed in suitable containers ready for the doctor to carry to his surgery for detailed examination. Pearce had already formed the suspicion that Charley had been poisoned so he applied the ammonia nitrate of silver test to the organs. The results, although not decisive, were enough to cause concern, so he meticulously packed all the organs into four flasks, which he sealed. These he gave to his servant to deliver to Mr Image in Bury St Edmunds for more detailed analysis.

Later in court the expert witness, Mr Image, identified the contents of the flasks he had received. The first was labelled 'contents of stomach'; the second was 'the stomach', the third 'urine'. The fourth, a 'pot tied & covered over' (presumably Mr Pearce's idea of 'sealing'), contained the bladder and its contents, the right lung, the right kidney, part of the right lobe of the liver with the gall bladder and its contents, the heart, the duodenum and the rectum. The specialist's analysis gave definitive evidence of arsenic in the stomach, with traces of the poison in the urine and minute traces in some of the other organs.

He explained to the court that arsenic would take immediate affect on an empty stomach but would take longer if it was in food. If the child had taken it on Sunday it would have taken effect before breakfast on Monday. He also volunteered the information that it was possible for arsenic to be placed on the lips of a sleeping child, in which case death would be between eighteen and thirty-six hours from its administration. It was also noted that seven-year-old David had had diarrhoea and vomited but he had recovered.

Addressing the jury, the coroner said that there was no doubt that Charley's death was from unnatural causes, that is, arsenic poisoning. This then posed the question, was the arsenic deliberately administered by any person wilfully and maliciously intending to cause the death of the child, or did the child take it accidentally? The coroner found it hard to believe that such a young child could have taken poison accidentally; if he had, 'would not the father or mother have said, "Why, we had poison on such a day and forgot it and the child must have got at that poison." But there was no evidence of arsenic on the premises – in fact it was denied.' He continued:

> … coupling that denial with the strong scientific testimony that death was the result of arsenic, it seems to me to criminally convict some person or other – who, we have not evidence to show at present. It appears to me that the poison must have been wilfully administered and if you are of that opinion I think you will be led to the conclusion that you must bring in a verdict that poison was wilfully administered and leave the magistrates to pursue further inquiry. If you think it accidental, you can return a verdict that the child died from arsenic but with no evidence of how it came into the system.

The jury needed only a few minutes' deliberation before they returned their finding, 'That the child died from arsenic wilfully administered but by whom there is no evidence to prove.'

After that it was inevitable that a second post-mortem and inquest should take place on Charley's brother James, who had died

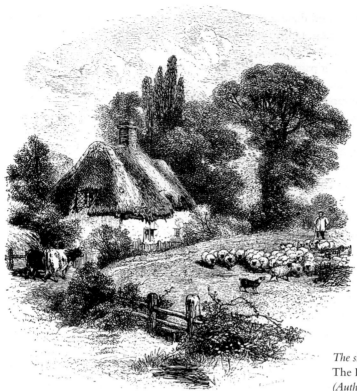

The shepherd at work. Taken from
The Infant's Magazine, *1877.*
(Author's collection)

at the end of June. There are no details as to who made up the jury for this inquest, which, like the first, was held at the Bell Inn, but the members certainly needed strong stomachs as part of their duty was to assemble in the church porch to view the newly-exhumed body. Although buried only some five or six weeks earlier, the cadaver was already in an advanced state of decomposition, in part no doubt due to the thin wood used for the coffin but also to the dampness of the churchyard.

For this second inquest, Sophia found herself under caution as a suspect. She related how, on the morning of Sunday 25 June, four-year-old James had complained of feeling unwell, in particular with an aching head. When this had continued, he had curled up beside the hearth. The family dinner that day was the usual boiled pudding and potatoes, of which James had had a little. But almost immediately he suffered a bout of diarrhoea, a situation that had continued for some time.

Being Sunday, Sophia did not send for the surgeon, believing that James's frequent bowel movements were merely indicative of an upset stomach. However she was worried about him and when she had looked carefully at his lips and inside his mouth she had noticed pearly white spots. So when her neighbour, Mrs Spear, called in during the afternoon, Sophia asked her if she thought he might have thrush. Elizabeth Spear, who had just spent the night sitting up with her own ailing son and daughter (both of whom were to die in the following month), noted that James's hands and arms were cold and clammy and that his face had a cold sweat on it. More worryingly, the child appeared only semi-conscious and his tongue lolled out of his mouth, around which there was white froth.

James's condition had worsened during the night and Sophia had sent her eldest son to Mr Pearce at four in the morning. Unfortunately, Pearce was not at home so Robert had explained the situation to Mr Ellis, his assistant, who gave him stomach powders and said he would call later. James died at half past seven, just a quarter of an hour before Mr Ellis arrived to examine him. By this time the whole family was suffering from diarrhoea, so Ellis dispensed more powders. To assist their recovery the vicar, the Revd Maul, sent them some brandy, which Sophia put into some freshly-made gruel. Fortunately, the rest of the family recovered.

The jury heard evidence from Richard Silver that James had been a sickly child and prone to fits. However, Elizabeth Spear attempted to cast doubt on Sophia's part in the deaths of both children by telling the coroner that after James died, Sophia had said she would lose another child within the month. When questioned about that, Sophia explained it was because she believed in an old country superstition. Their clock had stopped suddenly and been silent for some time, and then, just as suddenly, it had chimed, a sure sign of a forthcoming death.

Just when those in the village had made up their minds that Sophia Silver had done away with both of her children, doubt was cast on her guilt. The shepherd who had had his sheep in the field adjoining the family's garden came forward to disclose that he had recently dosed his flock. Everyone knew that the mixture used to treat the sheep contained arsenic. The shepherd also admitted that he had disposed of the empty bottles that had contained the poisonous mixture by simply throwing them in the ditch that divided the field from the garden.

The inquest was adjourned so that Mr Image could analyse the organs and two empty bottles of sheep dip. On 31 August he reported that whatever had been found in James's remains, they were not composed of any mineral poison. Detailed analysis had found traces of about 100 minute white granules in his stomach, which were also present in other organs, but these were, in Mr Image's opinion, likely to be fungal in origin. The conclusion was that James had not been poisoned with arsenic even though Charley had. So, when they looked again at the events which led up to the second death, it was concluded that the curious two-year-old had found the empty sheep dip bottles and tried to drink from them. An accidental death therefore, but one which, but for the evidence of the shepherd, might well have resulted in the conviction of his mother for murder.

APPENDIX

Churchwardens & Overseers Accounts – Great Glemham to Charles Clubbe.
[FC121/A4/1 Courtesy of Suffolk Record Office]

Expenses of trial of Wells v. Gooch.

June 16 1835. Instruction for Prosecution. 6/8d.
June 17 1835. Writing to Mr Keen of Farnham requesting him to attend & be bound for appearance of his apprentice & servant (to save expense of subpoena) but he declined doing so as the aforementioned had left him and latter only a daily servant. 3/6d.

June 23. Writing to King, surgeon of Saxmundham requesting him to send me a statement of evidence which it was understood he had collected from a witness who knew the prisoner & had seen her go into Mrs Wells's house on day the parcel was sent but it afterwards appeared that what King had been told upon the subject was incorrect. 3/6d.

Perusing and attentively considering the several depositions taken in the case for the purpose of determining whether any & what further evidence would be required on the trial of the prisoner. 6/8d.

10 July. Drawing instructions for Crown Office, subpoena for Samuel Wainwright and William Saunders being the only means of compelling their attendance to give evidence & copy for agent in London. 3/4d.
Writing to agent. 3/6d.
3 copies of subpoena. 3/-

21. Writing to Mr Keen requesting him to have the witnesses who were not bound over in attendance on 24 that I might subpoena them, also Mr Mills that I might at the same time arrange the manner of her going to the Assizes. 3/6d.

24. Journey to Farnham to serve subpoenas & arrange witness attendance but Mr Wainwright not there & Mr Keen having informed me that I should probably find him at his father's at Hazelwood journey to latter place & Mrs Wainwright informed me her son was gone out but that if I left the subpoena she would undertake for him to attend the Assizes & from there to Saxmundham to ascertain the state of health of Mrs Mills who pleaded her inability to take such a journey & attending Henry Freeman to ascertain her real condition & he thought she might undertake to go if there was no relapse by travelling to Ipswich one day & Bury the next & making the necessary arrangements & leaving money with Mr Freeman for her & serving her subpoena.
£2.0s.0d

Drawing account of expenses previous to commitment for examination & allowance by committing Magistrates & copy for their inspection. 5/-

Drawing certificate of allowance – fair copy for signature, attending Capt. Shafto explaining the items, & to obtain his signature. 6/8d.

Attending Mr Ling upon his bringing letter from Mr King enquiring if the attendance of Mr pretty was necessary & informing him it could not be dispensed with. 3/6d.

Writing in answer to letter received from Mr Stopher stating that it would be very inconvenient to him to attend & requesting a remittance of £5.0.0. 3/6d.

Letter & sending £1.0.0 to Samuel Wainwright to pay his expenses up & giving him full directions for his guidance. 3/6d.

Instruction for Brief. 13/4d.

Drawing the Brief for Counsel & Proofs – 12 ½ sheets when fair copied. £4.3s.4d.
Fair copy thereof for Counsel. £2.1s.8d.

Writing to Mr Johnson the gaoler requesting him to let the bonnet which the prisoner wore when committed be taken to Assizes. 3/6d.

28, 29, 30, 31. Journey to Bury to conduct Prosecution at Assizes – out 4 days. £8.0s.0d.
Attending Counsel to deliver Brief & Instructions. 6/8d.
Attending Clerk of Assizes to give instruction for the Indictment. 6/8d.
Attending Counsel several times in consultation at request of Clerk of Assizes to advise upon & settle form of Indictment some doubt occurring as to manner of charging the offence & afterwards on Mr Jones & Mr Byles' opinion. 13/4d.

29. Attending Court & the Prosecutrix & Witnesses upon being sworn in Court & from thence to Grand Jury room when a new Bill was found late in the afternoon & the judge fixed to take case first thing in the morning. 6/8d.

30. Attending Court & the prisoner, after a trial which occupied nearly the entire day, was found guilty & being recommended to mercy by the Jury on account of her being subject to fits & her disordered state of mind Mr Baron Parke directed her to be brought up again on the following day for judgement. 6/8d.

31. Attending Court when sentence of death was recorded against the Prisoner & Judge told her that in consequence of recommendation of Jury her life would probably be spared but that it would only be on condition she was removed from the country for the rest of her life & that she should suffer as severe a secondary punishment as the laws of this country would permit. 6/8d.

Making out account of expenses of prosecution & attending Clerk of Assizes to process order for same & afterwards on Mr Oakes, County Treasurer to obtain payment & on the several witnesses to settle with them and writing receipts etc. 13/4d.

Total £23.7.6.

Payments made by Mr Clubbe

Paid: Justices' Clerk fees as allowed by magistrates Certificate.	£3.8s.0d.
For Magistrates room & expenses.	7/6d.
Edward Kell Constable of Bruisyard for apprehending the prisoner & keeping her in custody several days.	£1.8s.0d.
Stephen Leek Constable of Framlingham for journey & expenses to Saxmundham to procure the attendance of Mary Mills a material witness.	4/2d.
Crown office subpoena for attendance of Samuel Wainwright & William Saunders who on account of their being under age could not be bound by Recognizances.	6/-
Agents charge in London for attending Crown office to bespeak & procure subpoena.	6/8d.
Postage of letters to Agents for subpoenas & double postage from them enclosing same.	2/2d.
Horse & gig hire on journey to Farnham & Hazelwood to serve Wainwright & Saunders subpoena & thence to Saxmundham to ascertain state of Mrs Mills health.	13/3d.
Fee to Mr Byles with Brief & Clerk.	£3.5s.6d.
Crier swearing witnesses to Bailiff.	18/-
Fee to Clerk of Assizes.	£1.13s.6d.
Expense of going to, being at & returning from Bury 4 days.	£4.4s.3d.
Mr King surgeon of Saxmundham for own & assistant's & apprentice's journey to Framlingham & to Assizes & chemist's charges in London of 2 guineas for analysing cake being the sum allowed by order of the Court.	£29.2s.6d.
Jane Wells for her journeys to Framlingham & Assizes.	£4.11s.0d.
John Fisk of Bruisyard a witness.	£3.18s.6d.
Mrs Mills & Benjamin Mills her husband of Saxmundham.	£6.18s.6d.
Mary Stopher of Saxmundham.	£5.9s.0d.
William Stopher of Saxmundham.	£5.9s.0d.
William Saunders of Farnham.	£4.11s.0d.
Samuel Wainwright of Hazelwood.	£4.18s.6d.
John Baldry of Bruisyard.	£3.16s.6d.
James Malster of Bruisyard.	£3.18s.6d.
Various postages & expenses.	7/6d.
Total payments.	£92.9s.6d.
Mr Clubbe's Bill.	£23.1s.0d.
	£115.17.0.
Costs allowed by Court.	£89.16.0.
Balance to Mr Clubbe.	£26.1.0.

REFERENCES & SOURCES

NEWSPAPERS

The Ipswich Journal
The Suffolk Chronicle
The Bury & Norwich Post

BOOKS

Lane, Joan, *A Social History of Medicine: Health, Healing and Disease in England*, 1756–1950 (Routledge; London, 2001)
Wright, Pip, *Death Recorded: Capital Punishment in Suffolk* (Pawprint Publishing, 2006)

OTHER

Census Records for 1841, 1851, 1861
Coroners Records for the Liberty of St Ethelberta
Foxearth and District Local History Society
Ipswich Gaol Records
Memoirs of Richard Stopher – unpublished MS, Suffolk Record Office
Orridge, John, *Description of the gaol at Bury St Edmunds*
Parish Records – marriage, baptism & burial registers
Woodbridge Gaol Records
Zwanenberg & Cockayne (ed.), *Suffolk Medical Biographies*

Other titles published by The History Press

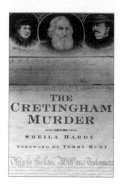

The Cretingham Murder
SHEILA HARDY

During renovation work on a hunting lodge near Aldeburgh, Suffolk, in 1996, a carpenter uncovered a plank of wood revealing a chilling pencilled message: 'A fearful murder was committed the first day of this month (October 1887) at Cretingham. A curate cut the vicar's throat at 12 o'clock at night.' From this strange beginning Sheila Hardy set out to discover the truth of this claim. It is a tale of religion and influence, politics and social power, mystery and intrigue, and is sure to appeal to all those interested in the shady side of Suffolk's history.

978 0 7524 4895 4

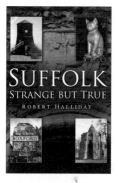

Suffolk: Strange but True
ROBERT HALLIDAY

In this book we discover the truth about the fasting woman of Shottisham, who was alleged not to have eaten for three months; the tithe war of the 1930s, when some farmers were reduced to selling their tractors for sixpence; unusual entrepreneurs, misers and witches, and also the tales behind a number of the county's deserted towns and villages. Local folklore and legend are also examined to show how real events have been exaggerated and embroidered over the years. Robert Halliday tells an entertaining story and alternative history of Suffolk that will fascinate residents and visitors alike.

978 0 7509 4704 6

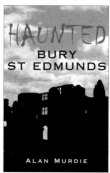

Haunted Bury St Edmunds
ALAN MURDIE

This book is based on spooky stories based on life-long traditions which have been handed down from earlier generations. Belief in the power of God and St Edmund still has a strong resonance in the town and reverberates across time into the twenty-first century. Against this backdrop, Bury St Edmunds may be considered a haunted area both metaphorically and literally and the book gives a comprehensive summary of the spectral residents of the town and its environs, preserving a permanent record of eerie experiences and beliefs.

978 0 7524 4204 4

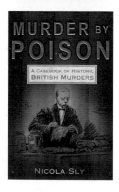

Murder by Poison: A Casebook of Historic British Murders
NICOLA SLY

Readily obtainable and almost undetectable prior to advances in forensic science during the twentieth century, poison was considered the ideal method of murder. While there are indeed many infamous female poisoners, such as Mary Ann Cotton, who is believed to have claimed at least twenty victims between 1852 and 1872, there are also many men who chose poison as their preferred means to a deadly end. Along with the most notorious cases of murder by poison in the country, this book also features many of the cases that did not make national headlines, examining the methods, motives and real stories of the perpetrators and as well as their victims.

978 0 7524 5065 0

Visit our website and discover thousands of other History Press books.

www.thehistorypress.co.uk